Ethics in
Nursing Practice

For Baillière Tindall

Senior commissioning editor: Jacqueline Curthoys
Project manager: Ewan Halley
Project development editor: Pat Miller
Project controller: Jane Shanks
Sales promotion executive: Hilary Brown

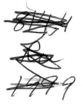

Ethics in Nursing Practice

Third Edition

Graham Rumbold

MSc, BA, RN, NDN, CHNT, DNT, RNT
Coordinator of International Affairs and
Continuing Professional Development,
Centre for Healthcare Education,
Nene – University College Northampton

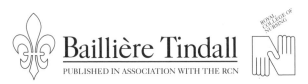

Baillière Tindall

PUBLISHED IN ASSOCIATION WITH THE RCN

Edinburgh   London   New York   Philadelphia   Sydney   Toronto

BAILLIÈRE TINDALL
An imprint of Harcourt Brace and Company Limited

Baillière Tindall, 24–28 Oval Road, London NW1 7DX, UK
The Curtis Center, Independence Square West, Philadelphia, PA 19106-3399, USA
Harcourt Brace and Company, 55 Horner Avenue, Toronto, Ontario, M8Z 4X6, Canada
Harcourt Brace and Company, Robert Stevenson House, 1–3 Baxter's Place, Leith Walk, Edinburgh EH1 3AF, UK
Harcourt Brace and Company – Australia, 30–52 Smidmore Street, Marrickville, NSW 2204, Australia
Harcourt Brace and Company – Japan, Ichibancho Central Building, 22-1 Ichibancho, Chiyodaku, Tokyo 102, Japan

First published 1986
Second edition 1993
Third edition 1999

ISBN 0 7020 2312 4

British Library Cataloguing in Publication Data
A catalogue record for this book is available from the British Library.

Library of Congress Cataloging in Publication Data
A catalog record for this book is available from the Library of Congress.

Note
Medical knowledge is constantly changing. As new information becomes available, changes in treatment, procedures, equipment and the use of drugs become necessary. The author and the publishers have, as far as it is possible, taken care to ensure that the information given in this text is accurate and up-to-date. However, readers are strongly advised to confirm that the information, especially with regard to drug usage, complies with the latest legislation and standards of practice.

Printed in China
NPCC/01

Contents

Preface to the Third Edition

It is now 12 years since the first edition of this book was published. At that time there were few books written specifically about nursing ethics, and those were largely American. Since then there has been an increasing interest in nursing ethics, evidenced by the number of texts and articles written on the subject and the emergence of a journal devoted specifically to the subject.[1] One might then ask *is there anything more to be said?* I believe there is. Just as much as for centuries philosophers, theologians and ethicists have continued to debate and write about ethical issues in the broader context, so the debates within the sphere of health care in general and nursing in particular will continue to occupy the minds of both theorists and practitioners.

Since the publication of the first edition, and even since the publication of the second edition in 1993, much has changed. Nurse education has changed; in the United Kingdom the implementation of *Project 2000* saw a raising of the academic level of nurse education along with the move of schools of nursing and midwifery into higher education institutions, a development mirrored both before and since in many other countries. Along with this there has arisen a greater interest in the provision of ethics courses within both pre- and post-registration courses in nursing and midwifery. The theory and practice of nursing continues to develop. There is an ever increasing interest in the study of the philosophy and nature of nursing, and alongside this the practice of nursing continues to evolve – the advent of primary nursing, moves towards the *nurse practitioner* and increasing emphasis on evidence-based practice. These and other developments raise new ethical questions, and increase the need for nurses to be autonomous moral decision-makers. As a natural consequence of these developments in the theory and practice of nursing there has been an increasing interest in the exploration of the nature of nursing ehtics as something distinct from medial ethics.

Nursing cannot, of course, totally divorce itself from medicine nor from the social context in which it is practised. Developments in medicine and changes in the expectations society has of health care have implications for and pose new ethical issues for nurses. In the United Kingdom implementation of the internal market within health care, the creation of NHS trusts and GP fundholding, all of which may yet change again, create new ethical issues and dilemmas for nurses. So too do developments in medical science and the emergence of new diseases such as AIDS.

In writing this third edition I have attempted both to explore further some of the ethical issues and principles discussed in the first two editions and also to discuss some of the issues arising out of the changes mentioned above. Some chapters have been augmented to take into account these changes and developments, one new chapter has been included and one chapter, formerly entitled *Euthanasia,* has been significantly altered, as the new title – *Death and dying* – suggests, to include discussion of other issues related to the care of those at the end of life. The new chapter. Chapter 1 – *What is nursing ethics?* – seeks both to make clearer the nature of ethics and to explore the differences between medical and nursing ethics.

In this, as in the earlier editions, I do not seek to provide answers so much as to raise questions and, it is to be hoped, provide frameworks for the reader to arrive at some answers. To enable the reader to enter more fully into debate with the subject matter some of the chapters now conclude with case studies and questions for discussion. The material for these is drawn largely from the real world. Some cases are taken from the literature while others arise out of the author's own experience or from cases presented by students. As in the two earlier editions I remain indebted to colleagues and students for furnishing me with the raw material on which to base my discussion. While it is the very nature of ethical debate that there cannot and will not always be clear-cut answers to every question, there is little point in entering into the debate if either the questions raised do not arise out of lived experience or the theories cannot be applied to the practical situation. Inevitably the dabate will be ever on-going in nursing and health care as much as in all aspects of life, but the debating only becomes of value if it aids individuals in making decisions when confronted with real problems. My hope and intention in this book is therefore to provide the reader with the tools to do the job.

Graham Rumbold
1999

NOTE

1. Nursing Ethics – An International Journal for Health Care Professionals, published by Edward Arnold, was first published in March 1994.

1

What is nursing ethics?

This chapter explores a number of questions. It begins by addressing the question of what is meant by the word *ethics* and the relationships between ethics, morals and philosophy. It then goes on to address the question why health professionals should study ethics. The discussion then moves on to explore the relevance of traditional medical ethics to nursing, suggesting that nursing needs a distinct ethic of its own and what the nature of that ethic should be. The chapter concludes by asking the question 'can there be a universal nursing ethic?'

WHAT IS ETHICS?

At its most basic, the study of ethics is concerned with the meaning of such words as *right, wrong, good, bad, ought, duty.* It is concerned with the basis on which people, individually or collectively, decide that certain actions are right or wrong, and whether one ought to do something or has a right to something. However, this is something of an over-simplification, for given this basic definition, one could legitimately substitute the words morals, values or mores for ethics. The question then is what does the study of ethics have to offer that differentiates it as an academic discipline?

> *Ethics … is a reflective, or theoretical business. It aims in the first instance at understanding rather than decision. … It steps back from the immediately practical and attempts to discover some underlying pattern or order in the immense variety of moral decisions and practices both of individuals and societies.*

> (Baelz, 1977)

Mores are the behaviours which a society determines to be acceptable behaviour. As such they are set in time and place, whereas ethics transcends the passage of time. *Morals* are often seen as being more concerned with practical rather than theoretical issues. '*Moral problems are*', according to Baelz (1977) '*first and foremost practical problems*.' However, as Baelz later points out, the distinction between ethics and morals is not clear cut. The words are often used interchangeably and given the same meaning, and strictly speaking they are interchangeable. The word *morals* comes from the Latin and the word *ethics* from the Greek and they originally meant much the same thing – '*the general area of the rights and wrongs, in theory and practice, of human behaviour.*' (Thompson *et al.*, 1983). Thus, many writers, including this one, use the words interchangeably. The reason being that, particularly when discussing applied ethics, that is ethics as applied to a particular situation or discipline such as nursing, it is inevitable that theoretical and practical problems become intertwined. For if ethics is to be of use to the practitioner in terms of providing a framework for decision-making it has to concern itself with practical problems.

What then distinguishes ethics or morals from philosophy? Here again the distinction is not as clear cut as, for example, the distinction between chemistry and physics. The two disciplines, ethics and philosophy, are closely interrelated, much in the same way as anatomy and physiology. Both philosophers and ethicists are concerned with finding meanings of abstract concepts and use similar thought processes and reasoning to try to find answers. And, just as students of anatomy and physiology might initially think they are studying the same things, so might students of ethics and philosophy. However, philosophy is concerned with finding meanings of a vast range of concepts. Philosophy is the pursuit of knowledge or wisdom, and especially that which deals with the ultimate reality. A philosopher might be as much concerned, on the one hand, with the question 'what is the meaning of life?', as, on the other hand, with questions such as 'why two plus two equals four' and 'whether truth telling is good or bad'.

Ethics is concerned with a more limited range of concepts. It is concerned with human actions and their effects and the value of those actions. These questions are also the concern of philosophers, but not everything that concerns philosophers is also of concern to the ethicist. Ethics then, is a branch of philosophy.

WHY SHOULD HEALTH PROFESSIONALS STUDY ETHICS?

The study of ethics seeks to provide means of formulating answers to questions and so guide actions. It provides a framework for dealing with issues, problems and dilemmas. An understanding of ethical or moral theories helps a person to decide on an appropriate line of action although it will not necessarily provide them with the answer. The study of ethics, while it may at first appear to be a largely theoretical exercise, does have practical application.

Nurses and others involved in the delivery of health care need to study ethics for several reasons. First, in their day-to-day work they have to deal with problems which are of a moral or ethical nature. Sometimes the ethical nature of the problem is very explicit, for example, when a nurse has to decide whether or not to tell a terminally ill patient the truth, or whether or not to participate in an abortion. At other times, the moral element may be less obvious, the decision on the face of it may be essentially a clinical one, and yet will be influenced, perhaps unconsciously, by a person's ethical beliefs and values. Health professionals need therefore to examine their own beliefs and values.

Second, advances in medical knowledge and technology have opened up possibilities which only 50 years ago were almost not thought of. Developments such as organ transplants, amniocentesis, *in vitro* fertilization, genetic engineering and criogenics, all raise ethical questions, the answers to which, are not readily to be found in any of the traditional moral codes.

A third reason is the changed world in which health care and nursing is undertaken. At one time it was probably fair to assume that there was a commonality of values and beliefs; that the values and beliefs of the individual nurse and patient would conform to the shared value system of society. In the United Kingdom, as in most of the Western world, that shared system of beliefs and values would be more or less Christian. We now live in a multi-cultural, multi-faith society and that assumption no longer holds. 'One of the major changes which seems to have taken place in our society during the last century is a shift from general agreement about moral values to what we now call moral pluralism.' (Thompson *et al.*, 1983). Nurses now find themselves working with patients and colleagues from a variety of cultural backgrounds who may hold very different sets of values. The nurse needs therefore to have an understanding of other belief systems in order to understand why individual patients and colleagues make particular choices. Later, it will be argued that two essential elements of nursing ethics are respect for autonomy and the nurse as patient's advocate. Nurses, if they are to respect the autonomy of others and develop the role of advocate, need to avoid imposing their own beliefs on others.

Finally, and perhaps the main reason, is the nature of health care itself. Seedhouse (1988) argues that 'work for health is a moral endeavour'. The essence of his argument is that the main purpose of health work is to enable the individual to achieve their fullest possible potential to enhance their own lives and the lives of others. This, Seedhouse claims, is as much the point of curing a person of their disease as it is of helping the 'incurable' come to terms with their condition. Health care is concerned with promoting, enhancing and maintaining health, and health is conceived as being morally good in itself. Health care is thus about attempting to create a moral good. This is very much a simplification of Seedhouse's argument, but it is sufficient to make the point that health care is of its very nature a moral activity.

THE DISTINCTIVE NATURE OF NURSING ETHICS

Historically, much that has been written about nursing ethics has been derived from traditional medical ethics. Before addressing the question of the nature of a distinctive nursing ethic, it is necessary to explore the main principles of traditional medical ethics and to identify their limitations when applied to the present-day nursing context. What will be argued here is that the traditional medical ethic derived from the Hippocratic tradition is no longer compatible with nursing philosophy, and that therefore nursing needs to formulate a distinctive ethic.

The traditional medical ethic

Traditional medical or biomedical ethics, at least in the Western world, are derived from Hippocratic principles. Central to the Hippocratic tradition are the notions of *beneficence* and *non-maleficence*, both of which are further discussed in Chapter 14. The Hippocratic Oath in its original form states:

> *I will follow that system of regimen which, according to my ability and judgement, I consider for the benefit of my patients, and abstain from whatever is deleterious and mischievous.*

In its more modern form (World Medical Association, 1948) this becomes:

> *The health and life of my patient will be my first consideration.*

From the above, it can clearly be seen that in its original form, the Hippocratic oath had strong overtones of paternalism: '*I* will follow that system ... which *I* consider for the benefit of *my* patients' (my emphases). And, even in the modernized version, the implication of paternalism is still there. The patient is seen as belonging to the doctor.

The point of contention is not with the principles of beneficence and non-maleficence. For no one could argue with the proposition that doctors and nurses have a duty to only act in ways which will benefit the patient and not cause them harm. The United Kingdom Central Council for Nurses, Midwives and Health Visitors' Code of Conduct (1992) states that nurses should 'Act always in such a way as to promote and safeguard the well-being and interests of patients/clients'. The contentious issues are who decides what benefits the patient, and how their best interests can be served.

It is argued that paternalism can be justified, and a much coined term is that of *beneficent paternalism*. We shall further explore this idea in Chapter 14. There are of course those who for various reasons are unable to make decisions for themselves, but they are a minority, and in such cases the doctor or nurse has to decide on their behalf what is in their best interests. However, paternalism, or to use Benjamin and Curtis' (1992) term *parentalism* 'means that an adult is being treated as if he or she were a child by persons acting as if they had the authority and concern of a parent'. In so doing,

Benjamin and Curtis contend, 'the nurse will claim to be acting on the behalf, although not at the behest, of the patient.' While there may be some justification for a parent acting in such a way with their child, 'Insofar as parentalistic coercion or manipulation of an adult involves a refusal to accept at face value the choices, wishes or action of an individual who is presumed to be autonomous and self-determining, it bears an even heavier burden of justification.' (Benjamin and Curtis, 1992).

The effect then of adopting the traditional medical ethic is to place the nurse in the position of parent *vis-à-vis* the patient. The patient becomes a passive recipient of care who is denied expression of autonomy. To deny persons their autonomy is to treat them as less than whole persons. The subject of autonomy is further explored in Chapters 14 and 15; here the main point to be made is that autonomy is an integral element of health. If a person is unable to exert their autonomy, for whatever reason, then they are not functioning as a whole person, and are therefore, if health is defined as wholeness, not healthy.

Seedhouse (1988) argues that if the definition of health implies autonomy, then health workers have a duty to create autonomy in the recipients of health care. The moral obligation of the nurse, or indeed all health workers, is thus to provide the patient with those things necessary to the expression of autonomy. This means removing those obstacles to the type of physical and mental potential needed to enhance people's ability to make autonomous decisions, and if necessary helping them develop the ability to make reasoned decisions. Seedhouse concludes that the creation of personal autonomy is the primary goal of health work.

Seedhouse (1988) goes on to argue that 'to respect autonomy is a major part of the core rationale of health work, and it is significantly different from the necessity to create autonomy.' Respecting a patient's autonomy means allowing them to make decisions and to have those decisions acted upon. Crucial to the ability to make autonomous decisions is possession of the necessary knowledge. This then places on the health professional a duty to ensure that the patient has all the information necessary to make a reasoned choice.

Attention needs to be drawn to the growing influence of the

human rights movement within health care. This has begun to manifest itself, particularly in the United States of America, but also elsewhere in the Western world, in the form of Patients' Rights Movements. The patients' rights movement argues that among the rights patients have are the right to be informed about all aspects of their care and the right to decide for themselves whether or not to accept health care, and when there are options which particular treatment to undergo. This is clearly in conflict with the traditional medical ethic of paternalistic beneficence.

The changing philosophy of nursing

The second strand of my argument that nursing needs to find a new ethic concerns the changing philosophy and role of nursing. The last four decades have seen the emergence of a wealth of nursing literature and development of nursing theories. While each theorist approaches the question of 'what is nursing' from a different perspective, and arrives at a different answer, there are common strands. Cameron-Traub (1991) states:

> *Threads in the evolution of nursing as a practice discipline are undoubtedly linked with philosophical perspectives on nursing practice and theory. Formal development of a body of nursing knowledge and theoretical expositions therein could hardly proceed without some degree of coherence in values and beliefs concerning the nature of nursing, what it is, and what it could (or should) be.*

Some of the common elements which emerge from recent theories are that nursing is about persons and human dignity, about acceptance of others, about holism, holistic health and holistic practice. Two key themes that emerge from the literature are that nursing is person oriented (as opposed to disease oriented) and that it is about helping people towards holistic living. The former means that nursing care has to be focused on the needs of patients as individuals and to respect their individuality. The second means that nurses are concerned with the whole person within the context of their life and environment, and not solely with that part of them which is diseased. It also implies enabling patients to exert control over their lives, that is to exert moral autonomy, for as I have already suggested, to not allow people to exert autonomy is to not treat them holistically.

Thus, it can be argued that while the principles of beneficence and non-maleficence are compatible with nursing philosophy, any notion of paternalism or parentalism is clearly not. The underlying philosophy of the nursing process and of most nursing models is that the relationship between nurse and patient is one of partnership not parent–child. The patient is encouraged to participate fully in all stages of the process. The nurse with the patient identifies their needs and plans their care. The patient is encouraged to participate fully in the implementation of their care, and the evaluation of the care received. The patient is thus actively involved in both the decision-making and treatment processes. An ethic which suggests that the nurse has the right to decide what is in the best interests of the patient is clearly at odds with the underlying philosophy of the nursing process and most nursing theories.

THE NURSE AS PATIENT'S ADVOCATE

Increasingly the nurse's role in relation to the patient is being seen as yet stronger than that of partner and rather that of advocate. The role of the nurse as patient's advocate is discussed more fully in Chapter 16; here it is touched upon to further illustrate the differing ethical positions of nurse and doctor. Why is advocacy so important? Because, 'without the advocacy and protection of rights, there are no rights. ... For the role of advocates is to safeguard clients against abuse and violation of their rights.' (Bandman & Bandman, 1990). If patients have rights, and I contend that they do, then if either their rights are denied them or they do not have the ability to exert those rights, the nurse has a responsibility to ensure that their rights are met.

This means that the nurse may have to defend the patient's autonomous decision even if she or he does not agree with the decision and if, as is more often the case, it conflicts with the opinion of the doctor or others involved in the care of the patient. The notion of the nurse as patient's advocate can, and frequently does, almost inevitably bring the nurse into direct conflict with the doctor. The conflict is not so much a clinical as an ethical one, for nurse and doctor often approach the situation from opposing ethical stances: the nurse from an ethical position which holds respect for autonomy as paramount and the doctor from one which holds that paternalism is justified in serving the patient's best interests when he or she rather than the patient has defined what are those best interests.

THE NURSE–DOCTOR RELATIONSHIP

The nurse–doctor relationship is undergoing change. And, although the change may appear radical to many, it has actually been a long evolving one. It began as far back as Florence Nightingale, who, although when she first arrived in the Crimea with her nurses forbade them to do anything to the patients until the doctors allowed them, nevertheless argued that nursing knowledge and practice were different from that of medicine. The evolutionary process which began in the last century has continued to this present day, and as has already been noted, there has been a tremendous growth in the development of nursing theories. As nursing evolves as a distinct profession, with a body of knowledge distinct from medicine, so the practice of nursing also becomes increasingly independent of the practice of medicine. Not least because the philosophical underpinning of nursing practice is quite different to that of medicine. Nurses no longer see themselves as handmaidens to the doctor but, at the very least, partners in care, and at best autonomous practitioners in their own right. It follows therefore, that as the profession develops a body *of* nursing knowledge rather than a body of knowledge *for* nursing borrowed from other disciplines, in particular that of medicine, then it needs also to discover its own ethic rather than be dominated by that of medicine.

THE NEW ETHIC

I have attempted to argue that nursing needs to discover a new ethic for three main reasons: first, the changing philosophy of health care with its increasing emphasis on the principle of personal autonomy; second, the changing philosophy of nursing with its emphasis on patient-oriented care; third, the evolution of nursing as a profession distinct from medicine. I contend that this new ethic therefore requires a total rejection of the concept of paternalism and, while retaining the spirit of beneficence and non-maleficence, needs to have as its main underpinning the principle of autonomy.

A UNIVERSAL NURSING ETHIC?

Much of the preceding argument could be criticised for its heavy Western overtones. The starting point of my argument was the Hippocratic tradition. Now, the Hippocratic tradition began with Hipocrates who was Greek and his teaching greatly influenced medical thinking initially throughout Europe and later throughout the New World. It has come to form the basis of thinking through-out what we now call the Western world. As we shall see in Chapter 3, thinking in other cultures is based on very different foundations. Thus, although the World Medical Association adopted a revized form of the Hippocratic Oath in 1948, there are long-standing tradi-tions in parts of the world which are quite different, and even in some parts of the world, particularly Eastern Europe, there have been more recent traditions which are not compatible with the Hippocratic tradition. Therefore, one might argue, if there is no uni-versal medical ethic how can there be a universal nursing ethic?

The nursing ethic which I proposed above is founded very much on the democratic principle of individual choice and rights. Now:

> *Applying ethical principles which build on the idea of democracy makes no sense in countries that do not have a political tradition that supports the respecting of patients' rights. Similarly, individualism (the cornerstone of western nursing) may often be inappropriate in a country where the concept of individual rights does not exist because each person must always act in the interest of the larger group.*

(Lutzen, 1997)

Lutzen argues a case for what she calls *context-sensitive frameworks for nursing ethics.* To support her argument she cites two examples.

The first is taken from a research study in Bangladesh and the second from an action research project to be undertaken in one of the states which made up part of the former Soviet Union.

In the first case it was the notion of informed consent which was problematic. First, it was not the participant in the research programme who was expected to be asked for consent, but another member of the family, despite the fact that the participants were adults. Second, difficulty was experienced in giving information about the study: 'When the researcher attempted to do this, she found it was not of interest' (Lutzen, 1997).

In the second case it was a range of issues arising out of the recent historical context, where nursing, including nursing education, is very much dominated by the medical profession, and discipline and respect for authority are the norm. The experiences cited by Lutzen correspond to those of the author when teaching in Poland. Ideas such as a negotiated curriculum and student participation, even the suggestion that nurse teachers themselves might be agents of change, were, initially at least, quite alien. The author's observation of practice in hospitals and health centres served to support Lutzen's view that concepts such as patient participation, autonomy, informed consent and respect for privacy do not form part of received thinking in cultures in which all are not perceived as being of equal worth.

However, this does not necessarily mean that the ethics of nursing itself should be different within different cultural contexts. What it does mean is that nurses moving from one culture to another need to be informed of the values and norms of the society into which they are moving. It does not mean that they should abandon their own ethical values. Nor, indeed does it mean that they should not try to impart those values to their professional colleagues in those other societies. For while it might be acceptable to argue that decisions about specific ethical problems might vary according to the individual situation, that one might not always take the same line of action in each situation, it is a very different thing to argue that ethical principles are context dependent.

If we accept the idea that every person is of equal value and that they should be respected as persons, then whatever the culture, whatever the time or place, they are still persons. The context does not alter the essence of what it is to be a human person. We cannot argue that different societal norms affect people's moral worth any more than they can change their biological make-up. Thus concepts of individual worth, respect for persons and autonomy are universal. That a society may deny people the right to be autonomous does not in itself mean they do not have that right.

To conclude, what is being argued here is that while a nursing ethic based on the principle of autonomy might have its roots in Western thought, just as does the Hippocratic tradition, that does not in itself mean that it cannot lay claim to universality. The reason being that people are persons, and personhood is the same whatever the context.

REFERENCES

Baelz, P. (1977) *Ethics and Belief.* London: Sheldon Press.

Bandman, E.L. & Bandman, D. (1990) *Nursing Ethics through the Life Span.* Englewood Cliffs, NJ: Prentice-Hall.

Benjamin, M. & Curtis, J. (1992) *Ethics in Nursing,* 3rd edn. New York: Oxford University Press.

Cameron-Traub, E. (1991) An evolving discipline. In Gray, G. & Pratt, R. (eds), *Towards a Discipline of Nursing.* Melbourne: Churchill Livingstone.

Gorovitz, S. *et al.* (1976) *Moral Problems in Medicine.* Englewood Cliffs, NJ: Prentice-Hall.

Lutzen, K. (1997) Nursing ethics into the next millenium: a context-sensitive approach for nursing ethics. *Nursing Ethics,* 4(3), 218–226

Seedhouse, D. (1988) *Ethics: the Heart of Health Care.* Chichester: J Wiley & Sons.

Thompson, I.E., Melia, K.M. & Boyd, K.M. (1983) *Nursing Ethics.* Edinburgh: Churchill Livingstone.

UKCC (United Kingdom Central Council for Nursing, Midwifery and Health Visiting) (1992) *Code of Professional Conduct for the Nurse, Midwife and Health Visitor, 3rd edn.* London: UKCC.

World Medical Association (1948) *Declaration of Geneva.* Geneva: WMA.

FURTHER READING

Gallagher, A. (1995) Medical and nursing ethics: never the twain? *Nursing Ethics,* 2(2), 95–101.

Kanne, M. (1994) Professional nurses should have their own ethics: the current status of nursing ethics in the Dutch curriculum. *Nursing Ethics,* 1(1), 25–34

2

What is right?

In the previous chapter it was stated that in part the study of ethics is concerned with determining what is right and what is wrong. This chapter further explores this question and will begin to discuss what determines whether particular actions are right, and if some actions are always right whatever the circumstances in which they occur.

Virginia Henderson (1977) gives as one of her components of basic nursing care 'helping the patient practise his religion or conform to his concept of right and wrong'. As noted in the previous chapter it can not be assumed, even within one social context, that nurses will share the same concept of right and wrong as at least the majority of their patients. It is no longer, if it ever was, the case that all nurses will share the same set of religious or moral values, and nor will their patients. Each individual's set of values will be the result of a multitude of factors, such as family mores, religious, cultural and educational background, and peer-group influences. Nurses as a professional group are divided in their opinions with regard to issues such as abortion, euthanasia and medical research. Views among nurses will range from those who would argue that abortion, for example, is wrong whatever the circumstances, through those who would say it is permissible in certain circumstances, to those who believe that every woman should have the right to have her pregnancy terminated on demand.

THE END JUSTIFIES THE MEANS

Contained within most moral codes, and certainly those of the major world religions, is the idea that to take human life, at least in most circumstances, is wrong. Equally it is a fairly generally held belief that to save life is right. It is, however, only a minority view that the taking of human life is wrong in all circumstances. Throughout history killing has been justified in certain situations, such as in war, as a punishment or as an act of mercy. Therefore, it would seem that it is not so much the act of killing itself that is held to be wrong as the reason for doing it. To kill an enemy during time of war is held to be justifiable because it is done not out of malice but for some good, the good being the protection of the State, the preservation of freedom and the protection of one's fellow countrymen. Similarly, the killing of criminals, in particular murderers, has been justified on the grounds that society thereby rids itself of evil and prevents the criminal from causing further harm to society or individuals within society. Mercy killing can be justified on the grounds that it prevents the recipient from suffering further pain. This latter issue is far more complex, and the subject of euthanasia will be discussed fully in Chapter 7.

What lies behind all these arguments is the idea that the end justifies the means. If the end result is a good one – for example, the protection of the State – then the means by which that end is achieved is also, if not good, at least justifiable and permissible. The implications of an ends-justifies-the-means philosophy are far-reaching, and not least within the bounds of nursing and medical practice. Such a philosophy could, for example, justify the experimental use of drugs on patients, which might be harmful to the individuals concerned, on the grounds that the ultimate end of such experiments was good: namely, to produce a cure for a particular disease and so prevent much suffering.

In Nazi Germany, doctors carried out a vast range of experiments on the inmates of concentration camps. Cancer was introduced into subjects and the progress of their agonizing deaths recorded. Others were stood naked for many hours in below-freezing temperatures; they were then warmed up to see at what points they showed vital life signs. Many died in the process and the remainder were usually killed afterwards. One of the Nazi scientists involved in these freezing experiments went to the United States after the war where he was to pioneer the development of American space medicine (Meltzer, 1975).

Suppose that the purpose of the first of these experiments was to discover a cure for cancer, and suppose further that a cure was in fact discovered as a direct result of them: would the experiments have been justified? The outcome would indeed have been of immense good; the suffering of many thousands in future generations would have been prevented. Suppose too, that as a direct result of the freezing experiments the scientist responsible was able to advance the development of space medicine beyond all reasonable expectations: would those experiments be justified? The answer of most people to these questions would probably be 'No'. Many would say that such acts were wrong in themselves regardless of the end.

The examples discussed so far are of a dramatic nature and do not form part of most people's everyday experiences. Let us now apply these arguments to less dramatic situations. Ask yourself whether you agree or disagree with the following statements:

1. To tell the truth is right.
2. One should tell the truth on all occasions.
3. There are occasions when to tell a lie is justified.

I cannot know your response to these statements, but I suspect that most readers would agree with the first statement, but that there would be debate about the other two.

Is it right or wrong to admire a friend's hat even if one thinks it terrible? It is something most of us have done at one time or another. In this case to tell the truth would cause the friend distress and may lead to an argument or further exchange of home truths. The end result of telling a lie is the happiness of the friend. No harm is done – or is it? The friend would no doubt continue to wear the hat and might make herself a laughing stock. Generally in such circumstances we couch our comments in words and phrases which, while not reflecting our true feelings, are not blatant untruths. We tend to call such statements 'white lies' and as such they are a generally accepted part of social interaction.

In the United Kingdom, as in most countries, when a person enters the witness box in a court of law they are required to swear an oath to the effect that the evidence they will give will be the truth, the whole truth and nothing but the truth. The very fact that in the special circumstances of a court of law one is required to take such an oath suggests that in normal day-to-day life people do not, nor are they expected to, tell the truth all the time.

Let us consider the following case. Susan and Jane are close friends. One day Susan tells Jane that she has been unfaithful to her husband, Bob. Susan asks Jane to tell no one, least of all Bob. What does Jane do? At this stage, having given Susan advice, perhaps suggesting that she ought to tell her husband, Jane is faced with a problem. Does she tell Bob or does she maintain silence? Her decision will depend on several factors: what she knows about Susan's and Bob's relationship, her own relationship with both Susan and Bob, and her own views on the rightness or wrongness of adultery. Jane may decide at this stage to remain silent on the grounds that Susan's unfaithfulness was a one-off event, and that to tell Bob would lead to more harm than good.

What, then, if two weeks later Jane meets Bob, he tells her that he suspects Susan of being unfaithful, and asks Jane if Susan has said anything to her? The problem is now more acute. It could be argued that to lie, to say she knows nothing, is justified. Firstly, the information was given her in confidence and therefore to tell would be breaking that confidence and could have harmful effects in terms of a lost friendship. Secondly, by denying all knowledge Jane might put Bob's fears at rest and prevent the possible break-up of the marriage. If, on the other hand, Bob later finds out that Jane has lied, this could lead to a loss of his friendship and the other consequences which she had tried to alleviate.

To tell the truth could have harmful effects, but might equally have beneficial effects. By telling the truth Jane might be able to explain the circumstances in which the act of unfaithfulness occurred and help Bob come to terms with the situation and thus save the marriage. Alternatively, he might react violently, return home and attack Susan, or walk out on her.

The problem we face when making decisions of this kind is that we can only hazard guesses at the possible outcomes. However good our intentions, we cannot predict or control the course of events. Proponents of an ends-justifies-the-means ethic would argue that if the intention is to effect a good end the means chosen is justified. Therefore if Jane lied to Bob in order to effect a good end then her action would be right, even if the end she tried to bring about did not occur. There is an inherent weakness in this line of argument. For a start it can be used to justify almost any kind of action, even those as extreme as the Nazi atrocities. We would do well to remember the old proverb: *The road to hell is paved with good intentions.* Secondly, we need to consider all the possible consequences of our actions.

If the deciding factor in judging whether an action is right or wrong is the intended consequences, then the criteria on which the decision is made are:

1. that the consequences are good or evil according to whether and how much they serve humane values; and
2. that the means to achieve those consequences are not so bad as to outweigh the goodness of the final outcome.

If the ultimate end is human happiness and well-being, but the means to achieving that end in itself creates unhappiness and suffering, which outweigh the goodness of the final result, the end cannot justify the means. For the end to justify the means the end itself has to be good, and a morally *good* end can justify a *bad* means on the principle of proportionate good. As we shall see in later chapters, this line of argument is used to justify such acts as abortion, euthanasia and deceiving a patient about his or her diagnosis.

PRINCIPLE OF DOUBLE EFFECT

There would be few who on reading about the Nazi atrocities would not react with horror and say 'No, such acts cannot be justified however good the end'. Such acts are, it would seem, held by most to be essentially wrong in themselves. Some would go still further and take a more absolute or purist view with regard to various acts. The pacifist, for example, would take the view that killing, whatever the circumstances, is wrong, because the act itself is wrong and cannot therefore be justified. What, then, if the refusal to do one wrong act results not in good but in further wrong? What if a man's refusal to kill a terrorist results in his own death and those of his wife and family? The result of his non-action is bad, although his motives in not acting were essentially good. The decision not to act is a moral or ethical one and can therefore be judged as being right or wrong just as a decision to act. A person does not abdicate moral judgement by doing nothing.

In situations such as this we have an example of what is described as the principle of double effect. In a situation in which to act will have undesirable consequences, and not to act will also have undesirable consequences, we have to weigh up whether to undertake the act. If the man does nothing the effect will almost inevitably be the death of himself and family. If he acts and kills the terrorist, assuming he is successful, then this too will have undesirable effects – the death of another human being, and feelings of guilt brought about by carrying out an act which he holds to be morally wrong. If he is unsuccessful in his attempt to kill the terrorist then in all probability the terrorist will kill him and his family. The end result will be the same as if he had done nothing.

In the earlier case discussed, Jane was faced with a similar dilemma – to tell or not to tell Bob of Susan's infidelity. The consequences of either course of action could be harmful. Jane's problem was, until confronted by Bob, considerably easier than that of the man faced with a terrorist. Jane at least had time to think, time to weigh up the consequences. Unfortunately, very often we do not have that luxury; the decision has to be made on the spot.

In making decisions of this kind there are four criteria which should be met, namely:

1. The act itself must be morally good, or at least neutral.
2. The purpose must be to achieve the good consequence, the bad consequence being only a side-effect.
3. The good effect must not be achieved by way of the bad, but both must result from the same act.
4. The bad result must not be so serious as to outweigh the advantage of a good result.

If the man decides to kill the terrorist, then (1) and (4) might give rise to debate. The question arises as to whether the act of killing can ever be morally good or even neutral. It could be argued in this case that it was neutral, for it could be argued that a man has a duty to protect his wife and family, and therefore if he refused to do so would be morally negligent. With regard to the fourth criterion, the bad result – the death of a person – could be argued to outweigh the advantage of a good result – the protection of wife and children. The problem of course is not that clear cut. For if the man chooses to avoid the bad result on the grounds that it outweighs the advantages of the good result, then the actual result will be bad – the death of several persons. His deciding not to act in order to avoid one bad result will have resulted in an even worse consequence.

There are many situations in medicine and nursing in which the doctor or nurse is faced with making decisions, and whichever decision is taken will have harmful consequences. Consider the situation in which a doctor is caring for a patient who is terminally ill and in severe pain. The doctor knows that the dosage of analgesia needed to relieve the pain is such that it will also hasten death. Death in such a case might be described as a side-effect of the treatment. It is clearly the doctor's duty to try to relieve the patient's pain. Not to give analgesia in order to avoid death, which is inevitable anyway, and leave the patient in agony would not be ethically defensible. Of the four criteria only the fourth might be an area for debate in this situation. The side-effect, death, might be considered to be so serious as to outweigh the advantages of a good result, pain relief. However, since death is inevitable, and will almost certainly be due to the disease, all that the doctor would be doing is making the process of dying easier and gentler for the patient. What it comes back to in the end is the consequence at which the act is aimed. The doctor is not aiming at the death of the patient, but at relief of his suffering.

NATURAL LAW

In most situations when faced with a moral dilemma people do not sit down and weigh up all the consequences. What in practice happens is that people act almost instinctively according to their own set of rules and values. Some people hold very firm views as to what constitutes right or wrong. Some, like the pacifist, would say that all that has to be considered is the rightness or wrongness of the act itself and not the circumstances in which it occurs, not the consequences of the act. It has been argued that just as there are natural laws governing the physical universe, such as the laws of gravity, so there are natural moral laws. If there is a natural moral law which determines what is morally right in any given situation it is binding on everyone and would therefore be absolute.

In Western theological systems, for example, which are monotheistic, God is the ultimate test of morality. Any action would be judged as being right or wrong according to whether it adhered to God's law. The question is, how can we know what is the divine law? Both Christianity and Judaism hold that the divine law has been revealed to man through his prophets and teachers, and, in the case of Christianity, through Christ. The account of God's revelation of his law are the scriptures. In addition, some Christian thinkers have argued that moral law can be discovered through the use of human reason.

It is not, however, only believers in these two religions who hold that there is a natural moral law. Indeed, it is not necessary to believe in any divine source of moral law to believe that a universal moral framework exists. This is true of the Stoics and of present-day secular natural law and natural rights theorists. The United Nations' *Declaration of Human Rights*, for example, states that every human being has certain rights, such as the rights to justice, freedom and 'a standard of living adequate for the health and well-being of himself'. Whereas those whose base for determining natural law is a theological one rely largely on revelation as the source of knowledge, non-theological-based thinking relies on reason, observation or intuition as ways of determining what is the natural law.

Immanuel Kant[1] argued that reason, or *practical reason* as he called it, can discover that there are certain rules of behaviour, or maxims, which become a universal law of nature. He argued that the way of determining if a moral principle or rule existed was to ask what the effects would be if it were to be applied universally. If the overall effect was good, then to behave in that way was right and in accordance with natural moral law. What would be the effect if everyone always told the truth? The effect would surely be one of universal good; therefore to tell the truth is a natural law. This is somewhat of a simplification of Kant's theory, but it does serve to illustrate how natural law can be arrived at through reason.

Others have held that the basis for moral judgement can be discovered by observation. According to this view, we are equipped with a moral capacity to sense what the laws of nature are.

Roderick Firth (1952), for example, argues that morality is absolutist in the sense of being independent of the observer. An action is right if it would produce a feeling of approval in an ideal observer, such an observer being one who is impeccably sensitive, impartial, consistent and dispassionate, but otherwise normal. Firth, and others, do not claim that such a person exists but merely that if he or she did we would hold as right anything which met with his or her approval. Firth says that in his ideal observer he has given what might be construed as a partial description of God. However, a belief in God or some other infinite being is not an intrinsic part of this moral standpoint.

If such an ideal observer does not exist we cannot, others have argued, determine definitely what his or her feelings would be. We have to rely in the end on our own feelings or intuition. The intuitionist holds that moral truths may be known to be true by intuition; that is, that they are if properly considered simply self-evident.

Whether natural law is discovered by revelation, reason, observation or intuition, those who hold that such a law does exist have a clear framework on which to base ethical decisions, and a set of clear and binding guidelines on which to make decisions. These guidelines could then be applied to all situations including nursing and medical ones. There would be no need for specific medical or nursing codes of ethics, for all one would need to do would be to refer to natural law.

If a patient reveals in confidence to a nurse or doctor an intention to commit a murder, the question is, should the nurse or doctor disclose this information. To do so will have the effect of preventing the patient from acting and save the life of the intended victim. In a situation such as this we should turn, not to any professional code of ethics, but to some framework which is more relevant to the problem at hand – to God's will or the natural law discovered by man's reason or through the moral senses. Thus the greater universal law that we should not take life and have a duty to save life would override any invented moral code which might hold that we should respect confidentiality or that the patient has a right to expect it.

While the concept of natural moral law has much to offer in

terms of making ethical decisions easier and more clear cut, it does have some weaknesses. We cannot be absolutely certain that we know what it is. This applies whether the basis is that of revelation, reason or observation. Throughout the centuries there has been argument about what has been revealed and how that revelation should be interpreted. People have reasoned differently from society to society and from age to age. Since no ideal observer is thought to exist, this school of thought relies heavily on man's moral sense, and the laws arrived at vary and are unreliable.

Probably the strongest argument against natural law theories is that acceptance of a universally binding rule removes the element of choice. Since I have the ability to reason and decide for myself what is right or wrong, not to use that reasoning ability would in itself be contrary to natural law.

Natural law is often invoked when discussing the question of contraception, for nowhere is natural law more assiduously applied than in the area of sexuality. Proponents of natural law say that God or nature intended sexual intercourse to result in pregnancy. To prevent the occurrence of pregnancy is to interfere with the natural course of events; it is to violate natural law and is therefore wrong. The question is: do we have the right to control events? If it is wrong to control the natural physiological process of conception, then it must equally be wrong to attempt to control other natural courses of events. We attempt to control many events that occur in nature; we build dikes and sea walls to prevent flooding and we build irrigation canals to prevent the formation of deserts. Is it any more or less moral to protect lives and homes by building flood barriers to control the rush of flood waters into a city such as London than to use a sheath to prevent the rush of spermatozoa to the womb? There is certainly a degree of illogicality in a line of thought which allows the one, but disallows the other.

The question arises as to whether the only purpose of human sexual intercourse is procreation. It is a fact that within each 28-day menstrual cycle conception is only probable during five to six days. Yet a woman's desire for sexual intercourse extends beyond that limited time. Unlike many other animals, human beings desire, are capable of and enjoy sexual intercourse at times when the woman is not fertile. Therefore it would seem that reproduction is only one purpose of sexual intercourse, and on the basis of time ratio relatively less important than pleasure. It is argued that another purpose of intercourse is an expression of love and affection; it is a means of communication. It is pleasurable because nature intended us to have intercourse for reasons other than the reproduction of the species.

Human beings are as they are as a result of the natural evolutionary process. That process has equipped us with the knowledge and ability to control our environment and our bodies. As a result we have a freedom of choice in being able amongst other things, to control our reproductive environment. It can be argued that exercising that choice is to exhibit a higher level of morality than leaving reproduction to chance. Since human beings have evolved to this stage, and since evolution is a natural process, not to use those evolved capabilities and to behave as if the possibility of control was not there would be against natural law.

The fact that we have the ability to do something does not of course make the doing of it right. We have the ability to destroy ourselves with nuclear weapons but it would be extremely difficult to justify doing so. There is a difference between preventing conception by unnatural means, and destroying ourselves and the world in which we live. In the first instance we are merely controlling one natural process in order to allow another natural process to proceed unhindered. In the second instance we would not be controlling a natural process but totally destroying the whole course of nature and not even replacing it with anything else.

We have the ability to reason and to make rational decisions. Not to use that ability, to act purely on the basis of a set of irrational rules, would be wrong. If using our ability to reason we conclude that contraception is wrong, then that is a morally mature decision, but so too would be to conclude that it was right. Either conclusion could be said to be in line with natural law.

SUMMARY

There is no easy answer to the question posed in the title of this chapter – *What is right?* Different people have put forward a variety of different ways of determining whether particular actions are right. One way of deciding is to consider the consequences; this I have called the *end-justifies-the-means ethic*. This idea forms an essential part of what is generally known as *utilitarianism*. There are different types of utilitarianism, of which possibly the best-known is that of Jeremy Bentham. Bentham and his disciple John Stuart Mill held that what determined whether an act was right or wrong was the extent to which it led to human happiness. It is from them that we get the phrase *the greatest happiness for the greatest number*. As we have seen, there are limitations to a line of argument based on either known or intended outcomes, and particularly where the outcome is merely hoped for but not known for certain.

The idea of natural law, while providing a framework on which to base ethical decisions, does not always meet the needs of the situation nor is it always easily discernible. What does one do when faced with a situation which is not covered by any known natural law?

In the following chapters we will examine further some of the questions and ideas raised in this chapter. We shall look at the influence of major world religions and ideologies on ethical thinking, and in particular what they have to say about natural or divine law. We shall return too to the idea that the end justifies the means and in particular consider whether the end aimed at should be the good of the community or society as a whole or the good of the individual. Other theories will be examined, such as duty-based and rights-based theories, and their contribution to determining what is right.

NOTE

1. Immanuel Kant, 1724–1804, was born of devout Christian parents in Königsberg, where he lived for his entire life. His interests were initially in the field of physical science, and it was not until quite late in life that he became interested in philosophy. In 1781, at the age of 57, he presented *The Critique of Pure Reason*. Other works followed such as *Groundwork of the Metaphysics of Morals* (1785) and *Critique of Practical Reason* (1788). At the heart of his thinking was the freedom of the

individual. It is, he argued, man's inner reasoning that dictates his moral actions. These actions, motivated by the mind's reasoning, are free actions, and it is this freedom that he must accord his fellow man regardless of status, colour or creed. Kant called this universal rule of action a 'categorical imperative'. 'Act only on that maxim that you will to be a universal law!' Kant stated the categorical imperative another way: 'So act as to treat humanity, whether in thine own person or in that of any other, in every case as an end withal, never as means only.' Kant died after a long illness in 1804, but his writings were to influence philosophers throughout the 19th century. Hegel and Marx drew on some of Kant's ideas in developing their systems of philosophy, and the existential ethics of Sartre and de Beauvoir in this century rely heavily on Kant's philosophy.

REFERENCES

Firth, R. (1952) Ethical absolutism and the ideal observer theory. *Philosophy and Phenomenological Research*, 12, 318–319.

Henderson, V. (1977) *Basic Principles of Nursing Care.* Geneva: ICN.

Meltzer, M. (1975) *Never to Forget: the Jews of the Holocaust.* New York: Harper & Row.

United Nations, *Declaration of Human Rights.*

FURTHER READING

Benjamin, M. & Curtis, J. (1981) *Ethics in Nursing.* New York: Oxford University Press.

See in particular Chapters 1 and 2 on 'Moral Dilemmas and Ethical Enquiry' and 'Unavoidable Topics in Ethical Enquiry'. This book adopts a case-study approach to ethical issues, applying various theories to the questions under discussion.

Fromer, M.J. (1981) *Ethical Issues in Health Care.* St Louis: C. V. Mosby.

See in particular references to 'utilitarianism' (p. 27) and 'natural law' (pp. 170–171).

Hursthouse, R. (1978) *Introduction to Philosophy.* Open University

Arts Foundation Course, A101, Units 13, 14 and 15. Milton Keynes: Open University Press.

See in particular Unit 14, Part 2, on utilitarianism.

Seedhouse, D. (1988) *Ethics: the Heart of Health Care.* Chichester: J. Wiley & Sons.

See Chapter 5, 'The Search for Morality' and Chapter 7, 'Therories of Ethics' for further discussion of the questions and issues raised in this chapter.

Warnock, G.J. (1967) (reprinted 1982) *Contemporary Moral Philosophy.* London: Macmillan.

See Chapter 2 for a useful introduction to the arguments surrounding 'intuitionism'.

3

Cultural influences on ethical decision-making

As we saw in the previous chapter, no two people will necessarily agree about the rights and wrongs of any particular action. There are several reasons for such differences of opinion. Our judgements are influenced by many different factors, not least the cultural background in which we live and have grown up. In this chapter I intend to examine some of the major ideological influences; namely, the Judaeo-Christian tradition, Islam, Hinduism and Marxism and a more recently emerging school of thought, commonly known as Western Secular Ethics. In just one chapter of a book it is obviously impossible to give a full account of any of these; each in itself would provide sufficient material for a whole book. I will therefore concentrate on those aspects of each tradition which have a bearing upon ethical issues in health care.

THE JUDAEO-CHRISTIAN TRADITION

Judaism and Christianity have much in common, much of Christian ethical teaching having its roots in Judaism. There are, however, some differences, and within Christianity some quite distinct differences between the two main traditions of Catholicism and Protestantism. Thus it is possible, and quite common, for Christians to disagree with one another about many ethical issues. I shall therefore attempt to outline firstly some of the key elements which are common to Judaism and Christianity and then those which are peculiar to each tradition.

The common core
The common core of Judaic and Christian ethical teaching is to be

found in that section of the Bible known by Christians as the Old Testament. Perhaps the best-known biblical ethical code is the Ten Commandments, though it is important to remember that the Ten Commandments form only a small part of the total picture. While the Ten Commandments are common to both Judaism and Christianity, the way in which they are interpreted varies. We already saw in Chapter 2 that the commandment 'not to kill' has been differently interpreted throughout the centuries. Furthermore, for the Jew, the Ten Commandments and other early ethical writings have to be viewed in the light of the Talmud,[1] and for the Christian in the light of the New Testament and subsequent Christian documents.

One thing that Judaism and Christianity have in common is a belief in the sanctity of life. Life is seen as a gift from God and therefore something which people should respect. Similarly, there is a belief in the authority of God, that there are God-given laws which should be adhered to. The debate is about how those laws should be interpreted and, particularly within the Christian Church, how God's law can be discerned. Nevertheless, there is for the Jew and the Christian a framework on which to base moral decision-making in life in general and in the specific area of medical ethics. Both traditions are frequently at variance with the Hippocratic tradition, which is of course neither Christian nor Judaic in its origins.

Judaism

The Jewish medical ethic is firmly interwoven into the religious tradition. It is not a professional code in the sense of a code drawn up by and for members of the medical profession. It is frequently given explanation and definition by the rabbis, who, while being extremely knowledgeable about Jewish theology and general moral teaching, may have little specific knowledge of medicine.

The essential elements of the medical ethic have been summed up by Jacobovits (1978) as follows: the sanctity and dignity of human life; the duty to preserve health; uncompromising opposition to superstition and irrational cures (including faith healing); a rigid code of dietary restraints and sexual morality; and strict instructions on the rights of the dead.

The emphasis placed on the value and sanctity of life cannot be overstated. Judaism totally rejects any compromise, including those of the Hippocratic and Christian traditions. No distinction is made between natural and artificial, ordinary and extraordinary, and heroic and non-heroic measures to preserve life (Rosner, 1979). So imperative is the injunction to preserve life that it takes precedence over almost all ritual commandments. Indeed, it is a moral duty to disregard ritual laws when they conflict with immediate claims of life or health. 'It is religious precept to desecrate the Sabbath for any person afflicted with an illness' (*Orah Hayim* 2: 338). The only laws which remain inviolate are those prohibiting idolatry, incest, adultery and murder.

To take life is wrong, as too is any act which might hasten death. The Jewish physician is bound to always strive to preserve life. To withdraw treatment from a patient who is dying is generally held to be wrong, although there is some debate about this. The Jewish rabbinic tradition recognizes a state called *gesisah*. This is defined as a stage in which the patient has become moribund and death is imminent. At this stage it is permitted to withdraw an impediment to dying. There is argument as to whether medical therapies which prolong dying can be considered as hindrances to dying.

Not only is it the duty of the physician to preserve life. The obligation extends to the patient. The patient has a duty to preserve his or her own life and does not therefore have the right to refuse life-preserving treatment, from which it follows that an individual would be acting wrongly if he or she failed to seek medical treatment if there was good reason for suspecting the existence of a life-threatening disease.

A Jewess would, for example, be under a moral obligation to seek medical attention if she discovered a lump in her breast, and having done so would be morally bound to undergo whatever treatment the physician prescribed, provided such treatment was aimed at preserving life. Some Jewish authorities would go so far as to say that if a patient refused life-saving treatment then this should be forced upon him. The Jewish position is thus in dramatic contrast to that of the patients' rights movement, the latter becoming quite widely accepted in modern Western thinking.

Equally strong in Judaism is the duty to heal. This extends

responsibility of the physician to include not only situations which threaten life, loss of limbs or serious impairment of health, but also much less grave situations requiring medical intervention to relieve symptoms or promote well-being. This latter point is remarkable when, for the most part, the medical and nursing professions have only this century begun to lay emphasis on health promotion and prevention of ill health. For the Jew it has been a long-held moral duty.

The Judaic laws governing diet and sexual morality are well known. While to 20th-century liberal thinkers these rules may appear rigid, reactionary and even nonsensical, many of them are based on sound practical reason. The rules governing the slaughtering of animals and preparation of animal flesh for human consumption, for example, make sound sense when one remembers they were made by a people living in a very warm climate before the coming of refrigeration techniques. Meat prepared in this way would not turn bad so quickly. The strict code governing sexual morality would prevent unwanted pregnancies and the spread of sexually transmitted diseases. Such laws are too a natural progression from the main underlying belief in the sanctity of life and the duty to preserve life and promote well-being.

Since 1953 when the Israeli government passed the Anatomy and Pathology Law there has been, in Israel, a heated medical ethics debate, not over subjects which have caused controversy in other parts of the world (for example, such issues as euthanasia, abortion, contraception) but over postmortems. The argument is between Israeli physicians who seek to advance their knowledge from postmortem examinations and the Orthodox Rabbinate which is concerned to maintain the traditional Jewish respect for the corpse.

Traditional Jewish moral teaching places strong emphasis on care of the newly dead. This involves far more than rituals to be observed when laying out the body. In *Orthodox* Judaism the body is held to be divine property and not merely the physical remains from which the soul has departed. No one, neither the State, the medical profession nor any other human agent, has the right to use the body for any purpose. Thus, not only are postmortems prohibited but so too are organ transplants. This respect for the dead body seems now to be unique to Judaism, but for many centuries it influenced Christian moral thinking. The battle over postmortem examinations, which followed the 1953 Act in Israel, was fought in the Christian world in the 16th century. Still today some Christians might find it difficult, even impossible, to accept the idea of organ transplants.

Jewish moral law does allow this rule to be overridden in certain circumstances. The requirement to save life can overrule the rules governing the dead, just as it can most other moral rules. Thus an organ may be removed from a dead body to save the life of an identifiable sick person. There would be no question of allowing organs to be removed and kept on ice for use when needed. To the non-Jew this would seem to be a ridiculous contradiction. Rabbis will allow heart transplants to be performed, because the heart is going to a known sick person and the action is life-saving, but not allow corneal transplants, for these are seldom life-saving.

Catholicism

Catholic medical ethics are extremely complicated. Most people are probably aware of some general moral rules that exist within Catholic moral theology. The proscription of, for example, contraception, abortion and euthanasia is well known. However, the teaching is not that simple. Abortion in the course of certain life-saving treatments is permitted as an incidental effect; that is, when abortion of the fetus is not the goal. Acts which some would call euthanasia are also allowed. Catholic medical ethics are based on two main components: 'a set of principles derived from the more general theory of Catholic theology and a more problem-oriented set of rules and insights to help people make decisions about ethical problems. This second component is often called casuistry' (Veatch, 1981).

The central core of Catholic moral teaching is natural law, but it is a particular understanding of natural law. The natural law is God-given and can be discovered by man through the use of reason. This creates a problem in that, since human reason is imperfect, our knowledge can never be perfect. Natural law can, it is held, be reasoned from understanding inclinations. For example, people are inclined to procreate so it must be natural law that they should. It is also held that natural law is confirmed by divine revelation. Thomas Aquinas summed up natural law as 'good is to be done and promoted, and evil avoided'. From this generalized law are derived principles which help to provide answers to specific moral questions. There are five main principles.

1. Stewardship

Life is given by God and therefore belongs to God. No one is owner or master of their own body. Humans are stewards of their bodies; that is to say, they have a duty to care for their bodies and protect both body and soul, from which it follows that one has an obligation to seek medical aid when something goes wrong with that body. It also logically follows, though is frequently overlooked, that each has a responsibility not to behave in a way which will damage the body, and take appropriate action to prevent ill health. It could be argued from this principle that it is immoral to smoke. Certainly the Roman Catholic Church has always argued that excessive consumption of alcohol is wrong, and of course gluttony is one of the seven deadly sins.

2. Inviolability of human life

This second principle derives from the assumption on which the first is based. Since life belongs to God, it is sacred and inviolable. It has given rise to the idea of a right to life, but it does not indicate a right to surrender life. What it in fact means is that no one has the right to take my life and nor do I. Rights in Catholic thought are inalienable; they can neither be confiscated nor surrendered. From this principle are derived the specific rules about such acts as abortion, euthanasia and suicide. However, they are not all absolute rules – there are some limits. For example, Catholic moral theologians have argued that there is such a thing as a just war, or that to kill in self-defence is justified, and some that even capital punishment is justified. The reasoning behind this latter point is that the life being taken is not an innocent life and therefore the act can be said not to be murder, which is by definition the killing of the innocent.

It should be noted here that the basis of these first two

principles is totally at odds with modern Western secular ethics and the argument that 'it's my body anyway'.

3. Totality

Given that the body belongs to God, and is in effect only on loan to the individual, how can surgery be justified? Surely the logical deduction from the first two principles would be that any interference involving the removal, mutilation or destruction of part of the body must be wrong. The problem is overcome by the principle of *totality*, according to which each part only exists for the good of the whole. Thus if an organ is diseased and thereby endangering the whole it may be removed.

The principle applies only to the individual body. It cannot be extended to sacrificing an individual for the sake of society. It does not therefore justify experimentation on humans for the good of society, nor the removal of an organ from one person to another. Nor does it justify the removal of a live fetus from a mother in order to save the mother's life. Such an act would be the destruction of one human life for the sake of another.

4. Sexuality and procreation

Throughout its history, Christianity has had problems in coming to terms with sexuality and defining the function of marriage. St Paul was generally opposed to the idea of marriage, and the nearest he ever came to endorsing it was to say, 'It is better to marry than to burn' (1 Corinthians 7, 9).

In Catholic moral theology, marriage has two prime functions. The first is the procreation and nurturing of children, and the second, the expression of love between a man and a woman. Until recent years more emphasis has been placed on the first function than the second, the second being for the good of the individual while the first is 'primarily for the good of the species' (Kelly, 1958). Thus follows quite naturally the prohibition on sterilization and contraception.

What, then, if a woman has cancer of the uterus and the only way to save her life is by removing it? To do so would accord with the principle of totality but contravene the principle of sexuality and procreation. Strangely enough, Catholic moral theologians would justify removal of the uterus and do so even if the woman was pregnant. They would do so on the grounds of the fifth principle.

5. The principle of double effect

This principle, which has been discussed in Chapter 2, is one which many ordinary people have come to by intuition. Catholic moral theologians have 'taken this intuition to a point of scholarly precision and elegance' (Veatch, 1981). The circumstances that have to exist to justify what would normally be considered an immoral act have been discussed in the previous chapter. Here it is sufficient to point out that this principle allows Catholic thinkers to justify acts which would normally be proscribed by one or more of the other four principles.

In cases where there is debate or uncertainty recourse is to the authority of the Church.

Protestantism

Whereas Catholic ethics are complex, Protestant ethics, at least Protestant medical ethics, are vague. While Catholic ethics are based on clearly defined principles, Protestant ethics tend to rely on broad theological themes on which to base individual decisions. In the more general field of morals Protestantism does provide well-defined rules. These rules, such as those relating to sexual behaviour, murder and property, are based upon biblical teaching. When it comes to the more specific area of medical ethics there are no such rules, largely because the answers to the problems posed are not to be found in the Bible. To answer such questions Protestant ethicists refer to two theological themes which emerge from scripture – covenant and agape or love.

Covenant is based on an ethic of keeping promises. The idea of a covenant relationship can be traced back to the Old Testament. One of the main themes in Old Testament theology is that of the covenent relationship between God and his chosen people. Protestant theologians have extended this to encompass relationships between people, in particular between one member of the Body of Christ (the Church) and others, both individually and collectively. In becoming a member of the Church a person enters into a covenant relationship with God and with his fellow Christians. This imposes on him certain duties and obligations, in particular to be faithful and loyal. Some Protestant theologians have argued that this idea of a covenant relationship can be applied in all human relationships, including that of a professional with a lay person. There is debate as to whether the covenant relationship between doctor and patient is reciprocal or unilateral. Some would argue that while the doctor or other professional, having agreed to accept the patient or client, enters into a covenant or contract to benefit the patient or client, there is no reciprocal obligation on the part of the patient or client to do anything. Others have argued that the relationship, once entered into, binds both professional and client and imposes upon both certain duties and obligations. The professional is bound to benefit the client, the client is bound to accept the advice and instructions of the professional.

Agape or *love* is a central theme of all Christian theology. Ramsey (1970) refers to it as 'a moral quality of attitude and of action owed to all men by any man who steps into a covenant with another man'. The problem is in deciding what is the loving action in any given situation. Some, such as Fletcher (1981), have argued that the loving act is the one which will produce the best consequences, an idea which closely resembles that of Aquinas, of doing good and avoiding evil.

How can one decide what is the loving thing to do in any given situation? Take, for example, the case of a new-born child who is severely physically and mentally handicapped. It could be argued that the loving thing to do would be to actively assist in the child's death, thus sparing the parents much anguish and hardship in the long term and, although it is much more difficult to determine, saving the child from suffering. To do so would of course contravene the commandment not to kill, and may actually cause the parents to suffer anguish as a result of guilt feelings. What is impossible to be certain of is the degree, if any, of suffering that the child might undergo if allowed to live. The answer probably is that in such a situation whatever decision is taken would be judged on its motives and that neither would be condemned.

It should be pointed out, however, that although there is this strong inclination in Protestantism towards judging every case individually, there is no more question of giving authority for deciding medical ethics to the profession than there is in Judaism or Catholicism.

ISLAM

Islamic ethical teaching has been influenced by a number of other cultures, among them Greek, Jewish, Christian, Indian and Persian. Nevertheless, although strands of these various cultures can be detected, there is a distinct Muslim belief system. The summary of the Muslim faith, 'There is no god but Allah, and Muhammad is Allah's apostle', lies at the core of all Islamic ethical teaching. From this basic affirmation naturally stems the notion that in all things *Allah's will be done*. There is a certain fatalism about the Islamic approach to life. Whatever action humans take, including the skilled intervention of doctors and nurses, at the end of the day the outcome will be as preordained by Allah. If it is Allah's will that the patient recover then he will, with or without treatment, and if it is Allah's will that he die then he will, however skilled the physician.

This anti-interventionist attitude, which is never taken to the extreme of totally forbidding any kind of human intervention in the natural state of affairs, gives rise to objections to some medical procedures. Muslim ethicists raise strong objections to anatomical dissection and organ transplants, though partly on the grounds that they would have some effect on life after death. Birth control too creates a moral problem, not for the same reasons as in Catholicism but because fertility is generally viewed as being something which is in the hands of Allah.

The following is a translation from the Koran by Pickthall (1953):

> *Whoever killeth a human being for other than manslaughter or corruption in the earth, it shall be as if he had killed all mankind, and whoso saveth the life of one, it shall be as if he had saved the life of all mankind.*

Thus actively ending the life of a handicapped child, as in the example given earlier, is strongly forbidden, as is euthanasia, and presumably so too would be assisting another by providing them with the necessary knowledge of how to do so.

This attitude of non-intervention linked to a fatalistic approach leads not surprisingly to quite contradictory views. Some Muslim authorities have argued, for example, that contraception is allowed, since fertility is in the hands of Allah, and so whether conception will result from coitus is determined by Allah and the use of contraceptive measures is irrelevant. Muhammad himself is reputed to have said of coitus interruptus (the major method of contraception at that time), 'Do as you please, whatever God has willed will happen, and not all semen result in children' (Musallam, 1978).

From this, one might be forgiven for deducing that Muslims are left either with permission to do almost anything, because whatever one does cannot effect the outcome, or with innumerable situations in which one cannot know how to act. Neither is in fact the case. Islamic teaching lays down some very firm and definite laws; for example, the prohibition on alcohol, laws relating to sexual morality and the rights and duties of individuals in relation to their superiors, especially of women to men. In cases where there is doubt or argument as to the morally right action, then recourse is to the religious authorities, and, as in Judaism, it is the religious authorities and not the physicians who rule on ethical issues in medicine.

HINDUISM

Hindu medical ethics predate Christian and Muslim ethics and can be traced back to the first millennium BC. Obviously the medical ethics of India today have been influenced by Western thought, but traditional themes still predominate.

The first such theme is the *doctrine of reincarnation*. It is held that one's condition in the present incarnation is the result of one's actions in a previous incarnation. This has implications for medical ethics. The *Caraka Samhita*, one of the earliest medical writings, includes a list of people whom the physician should not treat, including those who are extremely abnormal, wicked, and of miserable character and conduct. The extremely abnormal would presumably include those with severe congenital handicap.

The second theme is the *proscription against killing*. While the

Caraka forbade the treatment of patients on the point of death (cf. the Jewish notion of *gesisah*), there is in Hinduism a great respect for life. Active euthanasia is most definitely ruled out.

A third, and perhaps most important, theme is the principle of *ahimsa*, which incorporates the notion of non-violence and even the concept of non-hatred. The adoption of *ahimsa* into central Indian thought is partly due to Buddhism, and has also begun to influence Western thinking. It requires the physician to place more importance on preventing harm than doing good. Non-intervention is justified on the grounds of non-violence, even if intervention may lead to benefit. Thus to take the life of a patient in order to relieve even the most extreme suffering would be wrong, because to take part in the violence of killing is wrong whatever the circumstances. Less dramatically, it would justify non-intervention in the case of an 81-year-old diabetic with a gangrenous toe. Amputation would bring the potential benefit of delaying the patient's death, but would in itself be harmful and cause potential suffering. Not to amputate would be in accord with the notion of non-violence and also the maxim that to prevent suffering is more important than doing good. It could of course be argued that not amputating might lead to excruciating pain and therefore that amputation is justified on the grounds of preventing harm.

MARXISM

While in recent years we have seen the dissolution of the Communist states of Eastern Europe, we should not assume that Marxism as a philosophy is dead. There still remain Marxist states in other parts of the world, and Marxism itself has had and continues to have an influence on moral thinking generally.

Essentially, the Marxist ethic is one of the end-justifies-the-means category. What distinguishes Marxism from the other belief systems discussed in this chapter are: first, there is no belief in a supernatural deity, if there is a supreme authority it is the State; second – and here Marxism differs from both the religious theories and Western secular ethics – far less importance is attached to the individual.

Individuals are not important in themselves, but only in as much as they are part of the whole. What justifies actions is not the extent to which they benefit individuals, but the extent to which they serve the end of bringing about a socialist society (Rumbold, 1991).

Morality is not absolute or constant but changing, depending on the state of society. Thus in a Marxist or Communist state the ethics change depending on whether the country is in a pre-revolutionary, revolutionary or post-revolutionary situation. Yet a further code of ethics applies in a developing country. The overriding purpose and direction of the whole ethic is the building of a socialist society, and acts are not right or wrong in themselves except in so far as they serve that end. The State also has responsibilities towards its citizens. It has a duty to protect, care, and provide for its citizens, not out of a sense of benevolence, but because by so doing it will help to ensure the stability and functioning of the State. It is generally held that citizens have a moral and legal right to a free and comprehensive health care system, and that the State has a duty to provide this.

However, as we have seen in recent years as the communist states of Eastern Europe have collapsed and become more open to Western scrutiny, there have been tremendous variations in the quantity and quality of health care provided. In some there has been a very comprehensive health care system, in others the lack of even rudimentary care, and in others policies which most of us would hold to be immoral.

It is difficult too to be certain what the judgement would be on specific issues in health care. Rules tend to change from time to time and from place to place, depending on what is seen as best serving the interests of society. Hence in Czechoslovakia childhood immunizations were as good as compulsory. The rationale for this is quite logical, in that a population with lower risk factors for disease clearly serves the interests of the State. However, it goes against our notions of individual freedom. Similarly, on issues such as contraception and abortion, Marxists will vary in their views and consequently the policies of Marxist governments will vary. While Marxists would not have any religious objection to either contraception or abortion, they may base their views and policies on the interests of the State, in terms of whether the desired goal is population growth or control. Hence in Romania both contraception and abortion were prohibited, but in China both are encouraged by means of a policy which penalizes those families who have more than one child.

WESTERN SECULAR ETHICS

Central to all the schools of thought we have so far discussed is the idea that there is some source of moral authority. That source may be divine, as in the case of the religions, or the State, as in the case of Marxism. Western society for many years now has become at the same time both cosmopolitan and secularized. Thus it has become necessary to derive some general moral principles which are not aligned to any one specific belief system and do not acknowledge any divine authority. It would be impracticable to have a societal ethic which was based, for example, on Catholic principles, when only a minority of the population subscribe to that belief. Consequently, what has evolved, and it has been a gradual and natural evolution, is an ethical framework which allows each individual to live according to their beliefs, while at the same time ensuring that there are certain overarching principles which prevent one group from imposing their views on others.

One of the emphases in all the schools of thought we have so far discussed is that of duty. In modern Western thought the emphasis has shifted from duties to rights. Two closely linked ideas which emerge are those of *individual autonomy* and *individual rights*. It is on these two elements of modern Western thought that we shall concentrate, as they are of particular relevance to health care.

Individual autonomy

> *Autonomy (literally self-rule) is, in summary, the capacity to think, decide, and act on the basis of such thought and decision freely and independently and without, as it says in the British passport, let or hindrance*

> (Gillon, 1986)

Autonomy is not an invention of the modern philosophical mind. The ideas of individual autonomy, and respect for autonomy, can be traced back to the writings of both the early Utilitarians, such as J.S. Mill, and deontologists, such as Kant. However, in modern thinking, the principle of individual autonomy is linked to the notion of self-determination, and gives rise to the idea that people have freedom to choose. Thus they have freedom to choose whether to seek health care, and whether to accept it. It also implies that they, as masters of their own lives and bodies, may, provided they are of sound mind, refuse treatment – and do so even if that treatment is life-saving. This is clearly at odds with most of the ideas we have so far discussed, and, as we saw in Chapter 1, also with the Hippocratic tradition.

Rights

The notion of individual rights, at least to the extent that the secular ethic has taken it, is also equally at odds with most traditional schools of thought. 'I am not aware of a single document in the history of professional physician ethics before 1980 that so much as mentions rights' (Veatch, 1981). Rights do not exist in isolation, and, as we shall see in the next chapter, the extent to which an individual can exert their rights is inevitably restricted. However, the attempt to exert one's rights can give rise to conflict. The patient's right to refuse treatment, for example, can clearly be seen to be at odds with the health professional's perceived duty to act always in a way that will benefit the patient. We shall return to this particular area of conflict in Chapter 14, where the principles of *beneficence* and *respect for autonomy* are more fully discussed.

Although, as noted by Veatch, the idea of patient's rights is a relatively new one, it has in a very short space of time become a central theme of health-care ethics. Ideas such as the right of every individual to health care, the right of individuals to consent to treatment, the right to choose between alternative treatments, women's rights over their own bodies, have become part of everyday language. It has led, particularly in the United States, to a plethora of Bills of Rights.

SUMMARY

In this chapter I have attempted to outline some of the main ethical themes pertaining to the major world religions and philosophies. What begins to emerge from even so brief an account are some common and some divergent elements. In all but one of the schools of thought discussed in this chapter the authority from which moral guidelines and rules are drawn is outside or distinct from the individuals involved in the situation. For all the religions the authority is God or some spiritual authority which stands outside the world, and for Marxism it is the almost depersonalized State or Party. Whereas for the religions the rules are for the most part constant, though their interpretation may vary, for Marxism the rules themselves are subject to change. Even so, within each of the belief systems, an individual faced with a moral dilemma has recourse to some authority, either religious or party ethicists and philosophers, who can interpret the general rule as it applies to the situation.

Western secular ethics differs from the religious beliefs and Marxism, in that there is no definable source of authority. The authority, if anywhere, rests with the consensus view of society. However, even this is debatable, since the underlying thinking is that individuals are autonomous moral beings, and therefore have the right to determine their own moral actions. Nevertheless, there is some constraint, usually in terms of the extent to which one individual's moral decisions impinge upon the moral autonomy of others.

The four religions discussed in this chapter have in common a respect for individual human life which, although expressed differently and arrived at by different routes, leads to similarity of teaching in respect of specific issues. Marxism is often at variance with the religions over specific issues. One main reason for this is that, while there is respect for human life, it is more a respect for human life *en masse* rather than individually. The well-being of an individual may be secondary to the well-being of society.

Consider again the case of a new-born child with severe mental and physical handicaps. Possible responses to this situation might be as follows. None of the religions would consider the notion of taking deliberate steps to end the child's life. The Judaic ruling, and probably the Catholic ruling, would be that efforts should be made to keep the child alive. Protestant, Muslim and Hindu would probably all favour non-intervention, though for differing reasons – the Protestant, on the grounds that to take no action actively to end or preserve the child's life would be the most loving thing to do, but that the child should be given tender loving care; the Muslim, on the grounds that it is Allah's will whether the child should live or die; and the Hindu, on the basis that the child is as it is because of its conduct in a previous incarnation and so falls within the category of persons whom the physician should not treat. A Marxist could well justify deliberately ending the life of the child on the grounds that its survival would in no way benefit society, indeed would place an unnecessary strain on society's resources.

Any one of us might agree with any or none of these responses, and our response might coincide with that of a different religion or culture from our own. The reason is, of course, that most people arrive at moral decisions by their own reasoning processes and may be influenced unconsciously by schools of thought of which they have no formal knowledge, so interwoven have the cultures of East and West become.

NOTE

1. The Talmud is a compilation consisting of the Mishnah, or accepted body of traditional law, together with the subsequent discussions or traditions concerning it which arose in the Jewish 'schools'. There are two Talmuds: the Palestinian and the Babylonian. In common usage reference is usually made to the Babylonian, which is fuller than the Palestinian. It more or less acquired its present shape about AD 500.

REFERENCES

Aquinas, T. *Summa Theologica*, I-II, Q94, Art. 2, translated. In Gilbey, T. (ed.), *The Dominican Fathers of the English Province*. (1966) Cambridge: Black Friars.

Fletcher, J.F. cited in Veatch, R.M. (1981) *A Theory of Medical Ethics*. New York: Basic Books.

Gillon, R. (1986) *Philosophical Medical Ethics*. Chichester: J. Wiley & Sons.

Jacobovits, I. (1978) 'Judaism', *Encyclopedia of Bioethics*, Vol. 1, p. 792. New York: Free Press.

Kelly, G. (1958) *Medico-moral Problems*. St Louis: The Catholic Hospital Association of the US and Canada.

Musallam, B. (1978) 'Religious Traditions: Islamic', *Encyclopedia of Bioethics*, Vol. 3, pp. 1264–1269. New York: Free Press.

Orah Hayim, 2:338, cited in Jacobovits, I. (1959) *Jewish Medical Ethics*. New York: Bloch Publishing.

Pickthall, M.M. (1953) *The Meaning of the Glorious Koran: an Explanatory Translation*, ch. 5, v 32. New York: Mentor Books.

Ramsey, P. (1970) *The Patient as a Person*. New Haven: Yale University Press.

Rosner, F. (1979) The Jewish Attitude towards Euthanasia. In

Rosner, F. & Bleich, J.D. (eds), *Jewish Bioethics*. New York: Sanhedrin Press.

Rumbold, G. (1991) *Ethics in Nursing and Midwifery Practice*. London: Distance Learning Centre, South Bank Polytechnic.

Veatch, J.D. (1981) *A Theory of Medical Ethics*. New York: Basic Books.

FURTHER READING

Baelz, P. (1977) *Ethics and Belief*. London: Sheldon Press.

Jacobovits, I. (1959) *Jewish Medical Ethics*. New York: Bloch Publishing.

Kamenka, E. (1979) *Marxism and Ethics*. London: Macmillan.

Manson, T.W. (1960) *Ethics and the Gospel*. London: SCM.

Sampson, A.C.M. (1982) *The Neglected Ethic – Cultural and Religious Factors in the Care of Patients*. Maidenhead: McGraw-Hill.

Smith, W.C. (1962) *The Faith of Other Men*. New York: Mentor Books.

Reich, W.T. (ed.) (1978) *Encyclopedia of Bioethics*. New York: Free Press.

4

Sanctity of life versus quality of life

In this chapter two possibly contradictory positions are discussed; *sanctity of life* and *quality of life*. The implications of each for the provision of health care are explored and the question 'Can they be reconciled?' considered.

SANCTITY OF LIFE

As we began to see in the previous chapter, the notion of the sanctity of life is central to all religious or theological ethical codes. As Fromer (1981) states, 'the sanctity of life is related to the question of a divine presence'. If one believes in the existence of a divinity and that life is something which is given by that divinity, then one accepts the idea that individuals have no right to end life and a duty to preserve life. A rigid application of this notion would mean that in no circumstances should action be taken to end life and that in all situations every effort should be made to preserve it. However, as we have already seen, such a literal interpretation is adopted by a minority. Even within the Catholic tradition there is some room for manoeuvre, and in the other religious traditions exceptions are made.

Before looking at the questions to which a code of ethics based on the sanctity of life gives rise, it is useful to explore the notion itself in more detail.

The notion of sanctity

The first point to which we need address ourselves is the meaning in this context of *sanctity*. *The Concise Oxford Dictionary* definition of *sanctity* is 'saintliness; sacredness; inviolability'. The two words given that are relevant to this discussion are *sacredness* and *inviolability*. Anything which has sanctity is firstly sacred, that is to say holy and of the divine. It is something which therefore demands respect, even adulation. The problem is that all these words – *sanctity, sacred, holy* – are part of religious language. They have little meaning outside that context, and the concepts which they embody are only meaningful to those with a sense of the religious. They are totally meaningless to the person who has never encountered the religious.

Inviolability causes fewer problems inasmuch as it is meaningful to the religious and non-religious alike, though the two might disagree about the precise meaning of the word. For the religious, inviolability is closely associated with the notion of sacredness. Something which is inviolable is something which should not be profaned. A more general meaning of inviolable is *unbroken*. The religious might say that the laws of God are inviolable – they cannot or must not be broken. The non-religious might use the word when talking of the laws of the State. Thus to talk of the inviolability of life – that is to state that life is something which should not be destroyed – is not essentially a religious notion. It is not necessary to believe in a divinity to believe in the inviolability of life, whereas to talk of the *sanctity* of life, with its wider connotations of sacredness and holiness, is essentially a religious notion.

A phrase frequently used by ethicists and philosophers is *respect for persons*. Kant maintained that human beings should be treated as ends in themselves and never merely as means. The word *respect* is used here in an almost technical sense. It means 'that any person, as such, has intrinsic worth or value irrespective of his achievements, which, in the dealings of other persons with him, may be neither ignored or discounted' (Harris, 1966). Thus people of varying or no religious beliefs might unite in condemning the sort of experimentation on human beings described in Chapter 2 on the grounds that it was treating men and women as if they were not persons.

What life?

When we talk of the sanctity of life, what life are we talking about? Is it all life or some life? If we are solely concerned with human life then the question is what constitutes human life? Or if we talk about respect for persons, what is a person?

Some would argue that it is life itself, in whatever form, that is sacred. In Hinduism, for example, there is a strong respect for all forms of life and a repugnance about taking the life of any animal, even of the lower orders. There are those, including some who have no religious belief, who will eat no flesh because they feel that it is wrong to destroy life.

Generally speaking, when the phrase 'sanctity of life' is used, as, for example, within the context of health care, it refers to human life. The area of debate which remains is about what constitutes human life. The questions raised cover the whole life range, from the debate as to when the life form *in utero* can be said to be human, through how near *normal* the being should be, to the debate as to when does human life cease. The debate about life *in utero* will be dealt with in Chapter 8. The question which concerns us here is essentially about what distinguishes human life from other life forms. For the religious believer the answer is the soul or spirit. For the non-religious it is the ability to reason. Humans are different from the animals, even the most intelligent, because we have a spiritual component, or because we are capable of rational thought, or both of these elements.

Religious and non-religious agree that man's capability for rational thought distinguishes him from other life forms. A non-religious person might well argue that a being which, to all intents and purposes, looks like a human being but has lost or, in the case of congenital handicap, never had the ability to reason is not human. Its life is therefore not inviolable. The religious argument would be that although that particular attribute of humanness was missing, another essential element – namely, the spiritual – remains and therefore the life is still inviolable. The religious standpoint is quite categorical. A human being consists of three facets, *body, mind* and *spirit,* of which the most essential is the spirit. However deformed the body and however disturbed the mind, even if the mind be totally inactive, as long as the spirit remains it is still a human life and is sacred and inviolable. The spirit continues to live on when death occurs. If it were possible for the body to continue to live after the spirit had departed then it would no longer be human and therefore not inviolable. The belief is of course that the spirit or soul becomes dissociated from the body at the moment of death and it is impossible to conceive of a spiritless or soulless being.

The non-religious does not accept the existence of the spirit or the soul but sees the person, or, a term sometimes used, *personhood*, as comprising something quite different but no less complex:

> *The philosophical notion of a 'person', for example differs from the notion of mere 'human being'. In philosophical debates, 'person' usually refers to a human being who exhibits some level of rationality, sentience and the capacity to feel and experience sensations and express desires and wishes.*

> (Richardson and Webber, 1995)

To simply see a person in terms of mind and body is then to over-simplify the concept. Personhood encompasses a number of attributes apart from the physical and mental processes. These attributes include what we might call emotions – feelings and desires – and also a *self-conscious awareness* (Stinger, 1933) or *awareness of their existence over time* (Singleton and McLaren, 1995), *the ability of the being to value its life* which *implies a basic degree of autonomy* (Seedhouse, 1988) and the ability to reason and for rational thought. Of all these it is the latter which are to be found in all definitions and which seem to be the most essential elements. Not least, perhaps, because the ability to reason and for rational thought are to some extent more easily measured than some of the other attributes.

Thus, it is argued that once a being has lost those essential elements of personhood, and in particular a rational mind, then they cease to be a person. There is no compunction to preserve such a life. The emphasis is placed very much on the mind as opposed to the body, though some would argue that it is the combination of all the attributes of mind and body which makes a person, and severe physical deformity, just as much as a deformed mind, is a criterion for judging a life to be less than personhood.

So we begin to see that even though religious and non-religious might both lay claim to a belief that human life is inviolable they are nevertheless poles apart. For the religious, a life which is the product of human procreation is born with a soul and is by definition human. For the non-religious, even though a child be born to human parents it may be considered less than human if it does not possess the essential elements which constitute humanness. Judgements are being made about the quality of life.

QUALITY OF LIFE

The phrase 'quality of life' is much used in health care these days. Nurses frequently state that their aim in caring for a particular patient is 'to improve his or her quality of life' or 'to maintain his or her quality of life'. The problem is how can any of us really know what is another's quality of life? Any judgement we make is inevitably largely subjective. In effect, what we do is ask ourselves how we would feel if we had that particular physical disability. How would it affect our life? How would I feel if I could no longer remember things as well as I do now? How horrible it would be to have the mental ability of a six-year-old.

A person who has all his or her mental capacity but is severely physically disabled is able to judge his or her own quality of life. A person whose mind is malfunctioning may not be capable of such a judgement but, because of their condition, may be totally unaware of their own limitations. The child born with, for example, Down's syndrome might be judged by the onlooker to have a very poor quality of life. The child himself may be quite satisfied and contented. We can of course never really know since we are not able to get inside someone else and experience life as they do. The elderly person who is suffering from senile dementia has a quality of life which to the onlooker is very poor and by comparison with their previous state is greatly diminished. But again we cannot know what it is like to be that person, who of course cannot tell us. We do not always know if such people are aware of their condition or if they remember what their life was like in the past.

I don't feel my age – so my old age is not something that in itself can teach me anything. What does teach me something is the atti-

tude of others towards me. Old age is an aspect of me that others feel. They look at me and say 'that old codger' and they make themselves pleasant because I will die soon and they are respectful. My old age is in other people.

(Jean Paul Sartre at the age of 80)

Within a nursing context we need to find some criteria with which to measure a patient's quality of life. Several models are available to us: Virginia Henderson's 14 basic needs and Nancy Roper's 12 activities of daily living are two such models. These provide a basis for assessment of the patient's ability to cope with living and provide guidelines for deciding the intervention necessary to improve the quality of life. Thus when a nurse writes that the aim of nursing care is 'to improve the patient's quality of life', he or she can define this more specifically in terms of objectives based on such criteria. There is no suggestion in all this of moral decision-making. The nurse so far is attempting to make an objective measurement of a patient's quality of life in order to identify the most appropriate nursing intervention to improve or maintain that quality. If on the basis of the assessment the nurse was to make a decision about the *value* of intervening, then a moral element is introduced into the process.

Models such as the two to which reference has been made could be used to determine which lives are capable of being enhanced and which are not, and hence which lives warrant intervention and which do not. One could, for example, say that a person unable to meet less than a specified number of needs had a quality of life which was so poor as to render that person's life of little value. It should of course be pointed out that the originators of any of the models used in assessing nursing needs have never suggested that their models could or should be used in this way. I merely introduced them here to illustrate the difficulties involved in, firstly, assessing a person's quality of life and, secondly, making a judgement about the value of a life on such a basis.

In the practice of health-care delivery there are occasions when decisions have to be made where some criteria for measuring the quality of life are used. Consider the following examples.

Example 1

If there are two patients, each suffering from the same disease and requiring the same treatment, but there is only sufficient equipment or sufficient dosage of a drug for one, then a decision has to be made as to which patient should receive it and which should go untreated.

Example 2

Suppose you are a nurse in a small casualty department and you are the only nurse on duty when two casualties are brought in. Both need immediate life-saving treatment. You can only treat one at a time, and whichever you treat first the other will quite likely die or at least suffer some permanent disability.

The first situation is one which doctors frequently face, particularly in countries where resources are limited but also in more affluent countries, with regard to highly specialized and technological treatments, such as transplant surgery or renal dialysis. Usually in such situations there is time to think, time to weigh up various arguments. In the second situation the nurse does not have time; the decision has to be made quickly or both patients may die.

In trying to find solutions to these problems we begin by wanting to know more about the patients involved: their ages, marital status, whether they have children, what are their occupations, their levels of intelligence and so on. In other words, we want information which will enable us to make a comparison either between the quality of life each might have if treated or the contribution they might make to society. We are trying to place a value on them as individuals – the one with the higher score wins!

On a wider scale, similar decisions have to be made about groups within society. Given that resources are limited, those involved in health-care planning are faced with deciding which services for which groups should have priority. Do they spend x pounds on a heart transplant unit which will save a dozen or so lives a year, or spend that same sum on providing more general surgical units and so enable several hundred people to have hernias repaired? Do they spend more money on acute services at the expense of the elderly or mentally handicapped? These are all moral questions. However much we try to rationalize our answers, at the end of the day we are making judgements based on a set of values. In the choice between heart transplants and hernia repairs one could argue that treatments which are life-saving have a higher value than those which are aimed at improving the quality of life. In deciding between acute services and geriatric or mentally handicapped services the case is less clear cut. It comes down to making a generalized comparison of the relative quality of life of two or more groups of people. The resultant quality of life of the younger group following surgery is likely to be better than that of those in the other two groups, however much services are improved. It is, of course, not a fair comparison to make. It is based largely on assumption rather than scientific measurement. The issues of fairness and justice in health care will be more fully discussed in Chapter 13, where we shall examine one such measurement which has been developed – QALYs.

The problem is that (as suggested at the beginning of this section) one cannot know for certain what is the quality of life of another. Those who have the responsibility of making such decisions would fall mainly into the first category – that is, those likely to place demand on the acute services; some might fall into the second group (the elderly), but none into the third group (the mentally handicapped). Thus their judgement about what constitutes a good quality of life is clouded by their own expectations and experiences. As a young middle-aged and reasonably healthy man with full use of all my senses and faculties I consider my quality of life to be most satisfactory. If I were no longer able to read, enjoy music, communicate with others, move about or care for myself, then I suspect my quality of life would be much poorer. I *suspect* that such would be the case; I cannot *know* until, or if, I have the experience. Therefore, I can easily fall into the trap of suggesting that someone who cannot do or enjoy things I do and enjoy cannot have such a good quality of life. In fact, that other person might consider their quality of life to be more than satisfactory. Those things which are important to me may be of little or no importance to another.

To have some means of measuring quality of life can be of great value in determining health care but it can also be very dangerous. It is one thing to use it as a basis for deciding the most appropriate intervention; it is another to use it as a basis for deciding the comparative worth of individual lives. It becomes even more dangerous if used to determine whether the life is human or sub-human. The justification of the black slave trade – and it was justified by generations of churchmen and others – was that the African native was *sub-human*. It was even believed by some that he had no soul. Hitler and the Nazis justified their experimentation on, and extermination of, the mentally handicapped and Jews on just the same grounds. Because so much emphasis is placed on man's ability to rationalize, then it follows that reduction or loss of that ability renders the life of less worth; it may be not even human. As we shall see in Chapter 7, this line of argument is one of those used in defence of euthanasia.

CONTRADICTORY OR RECONCILABLE?

We now have to consider the question 'Can these two standpoints be reconciled?' At face value it would appear not. In the practice of health care to some extent they have to be. Occasions arise, albeit infrequently, when a decision has to be made between saving one life and another. The response of a person of the sanctity-of-life school would say that our nurse in the casualty department should make every effort to save both lives. Some would argue that if as a result both died no blame could be ascribed, because the intention was right and all possible effort was made to effect that intention. Others would say that it was better to save one life than none.

Let us assume that in reality the nurse has two choices: to do nothing, in which case both will die; or to attend to one patient. It is obviously difficult, if not impossible, to justify not treating either. The nurse is therefore left with the decision as to which patient to treat first, bearing in mind that meanwhile the other may well die. The nurse can make that decision on the basis of two ideas: either which patient has the higher possibility of survival, or which is likely to have the higher quality of life. If the former option is unclear then the nurse must resort to the second. Although the nurse may hold a very strong belief in the sanctity of life, the decision here must be based on quality of life. The example is of course a dramatic one; nevertheless it does serve to illustrate the point that the two notions can be reconciled.

The sanctity-of-life approach does not, as proponents of the quality-of-life ethic would suggest, deny the importance of the quality of life. The sanctity-of-life approach argues that the quality of all lives suffers if life itself becomes violable. Unless every human life is considered valuable because of its very existence then the quality of life itself is devalued. It is when questions arise as to whether or not to preserve a life that the two schools of thought may be at odds with each other.

SUMMARY

We have in this chapter explored two apparently contradictory standpoints. Both are valid and useful positions on which to base ethical decisions in health care, although both do have their limitations. Neither can provide all the answers and, as I have tried to show, they are not necessarily mutually exclusive.

One of the problems encountered if one tries to base all decisions solely on the notion of the sanctity of life has already been discussed; namely, how to make decisions between two or more lives. It has also been argued that if one pursues the idea rigidly then one may well be guilty of inhumanity. Hence the Catholic teaching on *extraordinary means* of treatment. The traditional stand has been that, while there is a moral duty to employ all ordinary means, one is quite justified in not employing extraordinary means. The problem today, with rapid advances in medical knowledge and treatment, is deciding what constitutes extraordinary means. Varga (1980) suggests the terms *useless* and *useful means* as being better for moral decision-making in health care. It would be quite in accordance with a belief in the sanctity of life to not employ useless means of treatment. I am not totally convinced that the terms *useless* and *useful* are appropriate in ethical decision-making. They are themselves value judgements and give rise to further questions.

If the notion of sanctity of life does not provide us with a basis for all decision-making, then nor does the quality of life. The major problem, as we have seen, is in determining what is the quality of life of another. If all the decision-making in health care were to be based on the notion of the quality of life, it is questionable whether many of the major advances of this century would ever have been made. 'Belief in the sanctity of life is the reason why health care exists and the reason why we are all concerned with the improvement of that care and its provision to all who want it' (Fromer, 1981).

It is probably reasonable to assume that most of the health-care systems which 20th-century man has inherited came into being at a time when there was a fairly generally held belief in the sanctity of life. The implication of Fromer's statement, which I would question, is that we owe health care solely to a belief in the sanctity of life, and that had the only belief been in the quality of life then there would be no health care. My own view is that a belief in the quality of life would have led to the inception of a health-care system, but that its scope and development would probably have been very different.

REFERENCES

Fromer, M.J. (1981) *Ethical Issues in Health Care*. St Louis: C.V. Mosby.

Harris, E.E. (1966) Respect for persons. In De George, R.T. (ed.) *Ethics and Society*. London: Macmillan.

Henderson, V. (1977) *Basic Principles of Nursing Care*. Geneva: ICN.

Richardson, J. & Webber, I. (1995) *Ethical Issues in Child Health Care*. London: Mosby.

Roper, N. (1976), cited in Roper, N., Logan, W.W. & Tierney, A.J. (1981) *Learning to Use the Process of Nursing*. London: Churchill Livingstone.

Seedhouse, D. (1988) *Ethics: the Heart of Health Care*. Chichester: J. Wiley & Sons.

Singer, P. (1933) *Practical Ethics*, 2nd edn. Cambridge: Cambridge University Press.

Singleton, J. & McLaren, S. (1995) *Ethical Foundations of Health Care – Responsibilities in Decision-Making*. London: Mosby.

Varga, A.C. (1980) *The Main Issues in Bioethics*. New York: Paulist Press.

FURTHER READING

Campbell, A.V. (1975) *Moral Dilemmas in Medicine*. Edinburgh: Churchill Livingstone.

See Chapter 5 on 'Respect for Persons'.

Fletcher, J.F. (1974) 'Four Indicators of Humanhood – the Enquiry Matures'. Hastings Centre Reports, Vol. 4, No. 6, pp. 4–7.

Schweitzer, A. (1970) *Reverence for Life*, translated by Fuller, R.H. London: SPCK.

Waddams, H. (1972) *A New Introduction to Moral Theology*. London: SCM.

See Chapter 9 on 'The Sanctity of Life'.

5

For the good of whom?

In earlier chapters the questions with which we were chiefly concerned were 'What is right?' and 'How do we know what is right?' The question which underlies the discussion in this chapter is 'Why should we do what is right?', or, put another way, 'Why be moral?' For some people the answer appears obvious: 'because God says so'. Alternatively, as was discussed in the latter part of Chapter 3, 'because the law, the State or some other authority says so'. These sorts of responses to the question 'Why be moral?' come generally within the school of thought known as *authoritarianism*.

Children who ask why they should behave in a certain way may be told by their parent, teacher or some other authority figure, 'Because I say so'. Such a response does not really answer the question, it merely begs further questions. Why do you – God, parent, teacher, government – say so? What is the purpose of behaving in this rather than that way?

At the risk of over-simplifying the various philosophical responses to these questions I have divided them into two groupings: those whose basis is individualistic – where the purpose is to benefit an individual, either self or others; and those whose basis is societal – where the purpose is to benefit all or a large proportion of mankind. Actions might be good because they serve self-interest, or the interests of others (*altruism*). The theories discussed in this chapter are all essentially *teleological* (from the Greek *telos*, meaning purpose) or goal-based theories.

SELF-INTEREST

One response to the question 'Why be moral?' might be to say 'Because to behave in accordance with what I consider to be right or moral will benefit me'. The benefit may be immediate – I will feel good, it gives me pleasure – or long term, such as in the next life.

One theory which judges the rightness or wrongness of acts in terms of an immediate or short-term reward is *hedonism*. Hedonism, as an ethical system, dates back to ancient Greece. Aristupus (*circa 435–circa 356* BC) is thought to have held that an act is good when it is capable of producing sense pleasure. Aristupus and his followers equated sense pleasure with happiness. According to the hedonists, happiness is the goal of man, and any act which brings one closer to that goal is good. Conversely, any act which causes pain or reduces happiness is morally bad. The early hedonists realized that a surfeit of sense pleasure is not necessarily a good thing; it may in fact cause pain and boredom. They were in no way condoning the excesses of pleasure-seeking, of drunkenness and debauchery which heralded the decline of the Greek and Roman empires. They recognized that moderation is the rule in all things and that it is a wise man who knows how to exercise sufficient control and avoid becoming a slave to pleasure.

Later Greek philosophers developed this theory further. Epicurus (341–270 BC), for example, also identified the goal of man with pleasure but emphasized rational rather than sense pleasures. Rational pleasures are those such as peace of mind, friendship and intellectual pleasures. Thus acts which increase these pleasures are morally good while those which do not, or prevent them, are morally bad. Aristotle (384–322 BC) advanced a similar view, and claimed that it pays to be courageous, generous or temperate because these types of behaviour alone give one a sense of happiness in one's relationships with others. A virtuous person is a happy person.

Consider for a moment how may times you have heard, perhaps used, such phrases as 'honesty pays', 'do as you would be done by' and other similar clichés. Why does honesty pay? Presumably because in the long run you will benefit by it, you will earn trust and respect and avoid getting into trouble – 'be sure your sins will find you out'. If you are kind and helpful to others then they in return are more likely to be kind and helpful to you.

The dishonest man may argue differently. He might say, 'Look where your honesty has got you; you are poor and taken advantage of by others, whereas my dishonesty has brought me wealth and power.' He might well conclude, 'Dishonesty obviously pays.' Provided his dishonesty is not discovered, and also bearing in mind that not all forms of dishonesty are illegal, he might go from birth to death without receiving any form of punishment. He might go on to say that he has no objection to others behaving dishonestly so long as in doing so they do not harm him. Thus 'do as you would be done by' or 'treat others as you would have them treat you' – what is known as the *Golden Rule* – while providing a convenient and practical guide to daily moral decision-making is not without criticism. It is based on the supposition that everyone has the same nature, the same needs and desires.

Most religious ethical codes are teleological and to a greater or lesser extent appeal to one's self-interest. The reward is not the immediate pleasure of the hedonists but something in the future. The promise for those who obey God's will is eternal life or, for those who believe in reincarnation, a better existence next time. The question asked of Jesus by the young man was 'Master, what good must I do to gain eternal life?' (Matthew 19, 16). The answer was 'Keep the commandments'. In the ensuing discussion the nature of the commandments and the moral behaviour that would bring about the reward was spelled out. There was no question that to seek eternal life was a right goal. The notion that the goal of morally good behaviour is eternal life is frequently emphasized in the ethical teaching of Jesus.[1]

There is a tradition of thought which is to be found in many religious and cultural traditions. This tradition holds that the human goal is self-fulfilment or self-realization. Any action which brings one closer to that goal is good, while any action which deflects from it is bad. This is as true of the early Christian hermits who sought a closer relationship with God as of the Buddhist monk, or the Hindu who leave their families to sit at the feet of a guru.

ALTRUISM

I am sure that many people reading the preceding paragraphs would say, 'That's not true. I am not kind to others in order to obtain some reward, I do it because I want to benefit them.' Or, 'I behave in this way because I will benefit mankind as a whole or the society in which I live.' This latter idea is sometimes referred to as *altruistic utilitarianism*, 'the moral idea for each agent to devote himself to the welfare of others at whatever cost to his own interests.' (Richardson and Webber, 1995).

Altruism (coming from the Latin *alter* – the other) is conduct aimed at the good of other persons. It is an integral component of many religious moral codes, not least Christianity where one is commanded not only to love one's neighbour as oneself but even to love one's enemies. Some exponents of a naturalistic ethic have agreed that altruistic behaviour has its foundation in the way things are. They do so on the basis that in the evolutionary process cooperation has proved more successful than competition. 'However, altruism usually runs so counter to man's self-regarding tendencies that it might seem almost unnatural.' (Macquarrie, 1967).

Many philosophers have argued that altruistic actions are always to some extent self-regarding; that they are done to earn esteem or the gratitude of the recipient(s), or simply to gain satisfaction from the feeling of doing good. While there may be some truth in this, it would be cynical in the extreme to argue that all altruistic behaviour is a form of disguised egoism. One can point to actions of individuals which have benefited others and have brought no benefit or reward to the agent themselves. Indeed, in some cases the agent has suffered harm as a result of their actions.

However, it would seem that purely altruistic acts are very rare. They would seem to occur more frequently within the sphere of individual ethics than in the context of social ethics. In fact, within the wider context pure altruism is probably never found at all. Reinhold Niebuhr (1965) argues that pure altruism is 'a moral ideal scarcely possible for the individual, and certainly not relevant to the morality of self regarding nations.'

Nevertheless, while pure altruism may rarely if ever exist, it is true to say that individuals' actions are not entirely motivated by self-regard; that people do act in order to benefit others. In the following sections we go on to explore further the idea of acting in order to benefit individuals and/or the wider social order.

FOR THE BENEFIT OF THE INDIVIDUAL

The response of many Christians to my earlier contention, that the reason for being kind, generous and caring to others is to inherit eternal life, might be that the reason for so acting is to demonstrate to those others the love of God and so bring them into the Kindgom. Similarly, a person with no religious conviction might argue that they behave in this way because they value that person as an individual, as a fellow human being. This leads to the maxim that in our relationships with others we should act in their best interests. The question then is who decides what is in another's best interest.

For the person with a strong religious or ideological conviction the answer might be that they *know* what is another's best interest or that the answer is to be found in the doctrine of their belief. The danger here is one of self-contradiction. For if one holds that each person is an individual, that they have an intrinsic value as an individual, and that they have the same ability as oneself to reason and choose, then by deciding for that person what is in their best interest is to deny them their individuality and value as a person. This was certainly the error committed by, for example, many churchmen and churchwomen in Victorian England. It gives rise, to a *paternalistic* approach which, until recent years, typified doctor–patient, doctor–nurse and nurse–patient relationships – the doctor/nurse knows best!

I used in describing this particular stance the word *error*, which is to make a value judgement. Not all would concur with my view that paternalism is a bad thing. 'I do not want to go along with a volunteer basis. I think a fellow should be compelled to become better and not let him use his discretion whether he wants to get smarter, more healthy or more honest' (General Hersley).

The notion of acting in such a way as to benefit others – *beneficence* – is a long-standing idea in medical ethics, having its roots in the teachings of Hippocrates. And, taken to its logical conclusion, it gives rise to the idea of *paternalistic beneficence* – the idea that someone, in the case of health care the doctor, knows what is best for the other person and therefore has a right to decide what they should do or what should be done to them. We shall discuss the arguments for and against such a stand in Chapter 14.

In recent years the trend in nursing has been away from *telling* the patient what is best for them and what they should do towards *involving* the patient in the decision-making process. It is inherent in the approach to nursing known as the *nursing process* that the patient, and their family, have a right to and should be encouraged to be involved in identifying their needs and planning the programme of care, and a right to make moral decisions. The philosophy which underlies the nursing process is:

◆ that people are individuals
◆ that, while recognizing certain basic human needs which are common to all, each individual has needs and problems which are peculiar to them
◆ that patients have rights over their own bodies and to have a say in what is done to and for them.

This naturally gives rise to what is sometimes described as individualized nursing care. From the patient's viewpoint this is doubtless a good thing, for no longer is he *a patient* who has had an appendectomy and therefore has known problems common to all patients following that operation and for which there are laid down nursing procedures, he is now *Mr Albert Brown*, aged 46 years, married with two children and employed as a bricklayer. He has a range of needs and problems, some of which he shares in common with others following an appendectomy but also some of which are peculiar to him because he is who he is. The nursing care can no longer be standard or routine but has to be planned for and with him.

Once we begin to consider patients as individual human beings then we have to accord them all the rights we accord to any human being and perhaps additional rights because they are patients. In recent years, the patients' rights movement has gathered momentum, and this has greatly affected not only nursing attitudes but also those of the other health professions. Rights-based theories and how rights are determined will be discussed in the next chapter. At this point what concerns us are the implications of the notion that patients have rights as patients.

One obvious implication is that the professionals are more likely to have their decisions questioned by patients. If this – as in many instances it has done – leads to the profession re-examining its own standards of practice, the body of knowledge on which its members have based their decisions and its values, then the effect must be for the better.

Another implication, perhaps less desirable, is that placing emphasis on the rights of the individual may lead to conflict. If there is one nurse to one patient or one doctor to one patient, then such statements as 'the patient has the right to considerate and respectful care' (American Hospital Association, 1972) present little difficulty. Indeed, there would probably be general agreement among nurses that all patients do have such a right. But what if the patient is one of 40 elderly men, many of whom are confused, noisy, demanding or incontinent, and there are just two nurses on duty for the night? Considerate and respectful care implies considering the patient's particular needs, taking into consideration that they are slow to understand or slow to move, respecting them as fellow human beings and paying them the common courtesy of stopping to listen to them. To afford all this to the patient in the first bed might be to deny it to the other 39. Therefore, the nurses have to make decisions about priorities. They have to decide which patients have priority and which needs of individual patients are more or less immediate.

There comes a point in all aspects of life when the needs and rights of the individual have to be considered in the light of the whole. Consider again the ward with 40 elderly patients and two nurses. Three patients have very definite and urgent needs, of which the two nurses are aware: Mr Jones has been incontinent of urine and needs a change of bedclothes; Mr Brown is in pain and has asked for his injection which is due – he also desperately needs to talk about his fears for the future (the two nurses being unaware of the latter need); Mr Smith is confused and noisy. There are obviously more ways than one of dealing with this situation.

It could be argued that the priority is to relieve Mr Brown of his pain, pain being a more acute and distressing problem than incontinence or restlessness. Giving an analgesic requires both nurses to be involved, one to administer it and the other to check it. It is not therefore possible for one nurse to deal with Mr Brown's problem while the other attends to Mr Jones or Mr Smith. In any case, both nurses will have to attend to the other two patients. Meanwhile, Mr Smith is becoming noisier and other patients are beginning to complain. If, when the nurse gives Mr Brown his injection, he pleads with her to stop and talk with him, the problem is compounded.

Another possible answer might be to say that Mr Smith should be attended to first, calmed down and given a sedative; otherwise he is going to disturb all the other patients.

FOR THE GOOD OF THE MAJORITY

Thus we begin to see that the needs of one person cannot in every situation be dealt with in isolation. Mr Brown was one of 40 patients, all with their own needs and all equally entitled to 'considerate and respectful care'. The nurses must apportion their time amongst all the patients. In such a situation it would seem more appropriate to attempt to meet some of the needs of all, rather than all the needs of some.

As we saw in Chapter 2 some utilitarians would argue that the main principle to be obeyed is to act in such a way as to give the greatest happiness to the greatest number. To some extent utilitarianism is a development and modification of hedonism, for utilitarianism accepts the notion that all people act to gain pleasure or to avoid pain. Jeremy Bentham (1748–1832) and his immediate followers equated pleasure with happiness, and said that the goal of human acts is to achieve the greatest possible happiness. The next step is to decide which acts increase happiness. These are then defined as good acts and those which produce pain are bad acts. Bentham called the property of the act that produces happiness *utility*, and hence *utilitarianism* is the name given to this particular ethical theory.

Bentham held that all pleasures can be *quantified* and that therefore it is possible to calculate the greatness of happiness. He argued that people are basically selfish but have necessarily to consider the happiness of others because they need the help of their fellow beings for their own happiness. Thus he deduced that the morally good act is that which produces the greatest happiness for the greatest number of people.

John Stuart Mill (1806–73), while accepting the basic principles of Bentham's theory, rejected the idea that all pleasures can be measured *quantitatively* and argued that pleasures differ *qualitatively*. Pleasures that befit rational human beings rather than those held in common with lesser animals have greater value. He also placed more emphasis on the social character of happiness than did Bentham. The goal of moral actions is the greatest happiness of all members of society.

Two further refinements of the utilitarian theory are *act utilitarianism* and *rule utilitarianism*. *Act utilitarianism* is so called because it is the act itself that is judged to be good or bad according to whether it serves the principle of greatest happiness. *Rule utilitarianism* tries to establish rules that are capable of producing the greatest happiness for the greatest number. The rules are arrived at by assessing the hypothetical consequences of everyone following a rule that a particular act is to be done or not done. For example, suppose I am a rule utilitarian and I want to decide whether it would be right or wrong to drop my empty drink carton in the street. What I do is ask myself what the consequences would be if everyone followed the rule 'Throw your litter in the street if you want to'. Or, more simply 'What if everyone did it?' The consequences would most certainly not promote happiness because the streets would soon become very untidy and hazardous. So the rule is not a right rule and therefore the act is not right. Rule utilitarians insist that rules are universally binding. Thus if the rule is 'to throw litter in the street is wrong' then no one is exempt from that rule. One person dropping one piece of litter in the street detracts from the cleanliness of the street and therefore from the greatest happiness.

There is therefore a fundamental difference between act and rule utilitarians, although both agree that the goal is the greatest happiness. Act utilitarians, because they judge each act by its consequences, may well judge an act to be right on one occasion but wrong on another. One would expect rule utilitarians to say that if the rule is that the act should not be done, then it is never justified whatever the circumstances. In practice, though, rule utilitarians are not so rigid – they do not hold all rules to be sacrosanct.

Consider, for example, the question of keeping promises. The rule is 'Keep promises'. Breaking promises is wrong because if everyone did so it would cause the whole institution of keeping promises to break down and that would certainly not promote the greatest happiness. Therefore one might think that rule utilitarians might claim that this rule is sacrosanct. Of course, to do so would be to afford to promise-keeping more importance than it deserves.

Suppose Jane has promised to meet her boyfriend outside the cinema at seven o'clock and further promised that for once she will not be late. On her way to the cinema Jane sees an accident – a small boy is knocked from his bicycle by a speeding car. The driver does not stop and the boy is lying in the road. He is crying and Jane can see blood on his face and hands. There is no one else around. What is the right thing for her to do?

An act utilitarian would have no hesitation in saying that Jane should stop and attend to the boy even though this means she will be late for her meeting and will therefore have broken her promise. If the rule 'Keep promises' were sacrosanct, then the rule utilitarian would have no option but to say, 'No, she should keep going and keep her promise'. That is obviously nonsense. Keeping a promise about meeting a friend is not as important as saving someone's life. The rule utilitarian's response would be to point out that 'Preserve life' is a good moral rule. Obviously, if everyone obeyed the rule it would increase human happiness. What he has to do in this case is to appeal directly to the greatest happiness principle, and clearly life-saving saving will lead to greater happiness than promise-keeping. In this particular case the act and rule utilitarians would be in agreement.

In providing a framework for moral decision-making, utilitarianism, and rule utilitarianism in particular, can be very useful. However, there is a flaw in the argument. Utilitarians base their argument on several suppositions. Firstly, they presuppose that everyone knows what the happiness or well-being of man is and that everyone understands it in the same way. If, as the utilitarians claim, everyone can estimate what actions promote happiness then each individual could set their own criterion of morality. The result would be chaos, which of course rule utilitarianism attempts to overcome. Another supposition is that everyone becomes happy in the same way – in other words, that acts which are anticipated to produce the greatest happiness will be pleasurable to individuals. Yet man's experience has shown that the best interests of the majority of people are not always served by such acts, nor do individuals always find their consequences pleasant.

The questions which, it can be argued, utilitarians have failed to answer satisfactorily are 'How can we know what happiness is?' and 'How can we determine the best way of achieving it?' Nevertheless, in some situations the notion of the greatest good or happiness for the greatest number can be a useful guide to decision-making.

In the example discussed earlier of the ward with 40 elderly patients this idea would enable the nurses to come quickly to a decision. The decision to deal first with Mr Smith would be a *right* one. In doing so, Mr Smith and 37 other patients in the ward would benefit. Quiet would ensue and they would be able to get to sleep. It would of course not meet the primary needs of Mr Brown and Mr Jones. So we come to another flaw in the utilitarian's argument; for in striving to attain the greatest good for the greatest number one might totally ignore or violate the interests of the minority and, in some cases, the minority might be quite a sizeable portion of the whole. The utilitarian's answer to this objection is that if the application of a rule had this effect then the rule would not be morally good because it would violate the fair and equal distribution of goods. In so doing utilitarians are contradicting the moral criterion of utilitarianism by appealing to a more fundamental standard, that of justice.

FOR THE GOOD OF ALL

In Chapter 3 we saw that in Marxist ethics the criterion by which acts are judged as right or wrong is the extent to which they serve the interests of the State. It could be argued, therefore, that the concern was not for the good of the majority but for the good of all, or at least the whole population of the State. So, on the face of it, Marxist ethics are aimed at achieving greater benefit than are utilitarian ethics. In practice, of course, 'for the good of the State' is not the same as 'for the good for all citizens', because what the Marxist is more concerned about is preserving the structure of the State rather than its contents. It may, for example, serve the best interests of the State to dispose of a section of the population. Certainly it means that there is no responsibility to act for the good of those outside the State.

The effect of applying Marxist ethics is to ignore totally individual needs and differences. It may lead, as does utilitarianism, to violating the interests of the minority, even those of the majority. Of course Marxist theorists would argue that in the long term anything which benefits the State will benefit the whole population, but the population it will benefit is in the future and not the present.

Is it possible then to talk of a code of ethics which seems at all times to benefit all? Some religious theorists would answer in the affirmative. Christians, for example, would argue that the ultimate goal is to bring all mankind into fellowship with God. What justifies any act is the extent to which it promotes that goal.

SUMMARY

In this chapter we have been concerned with teleological or consequential theories of ethics, where the criterion for moral decision-making is the effects or consequences arising from an act. Essentially, the various theories discussed can be divided, as I have done, into two categories: those whose consequence is individual good, and those whose consequence is the good of the majority. They could as well be divided into selfish and altruistic theories.

If one tries to base decisions in nursing or health care generally on the extent to which acts will benefit the individual, then this can lead to better patient care. It may, however, mean better care for one patient to the detriment of others. So while the growth of individualized patient care might be welcomed because it treats the patient as a person rather than as one of a number of cases, it may lead to conflict within the minds of the providers of care. If resources are limitless then there may be no problem. In practice, resources, including those of the individual carer as well as those of society, are limited. Care then has to be apportioned and priorities identified.

To base decisions on the criterion of the greatest good for the greatest number becomes a very attractive idea. It provides both the individual carer and policy-makers with a yardstick. However, as we have seen, it does have its flaws, primarily because it involves a large element of subjectivity.

In Chapter 13, we shall return to this issue, and explore other criteria on which judgements are made in determining who should receive what in terms of health care.

The underlying question which has concerned us in this chapter is 'Why be moral?' The theories discussed have all attempted to provide an answer, be it for benefit of self, of other individuals or of the greatest number. In the next chapter we will still be concerned with the same question, but will look at theories which attempt to answer it from a different starting point.

NOTE

1. See for example: Matthew 19, 27–29; Matthew 5, 1–10; Matthew 5, 17–19; Mark 12, 28–34; Luke 6, 20–23.

REFERENCES

American Hospital Association (1972) *Patients' Bill of Rights.* General Hersley, quoted in Dworkin, G. (1976) Paternalism. In Gorrovitz, S. *et al.* (eds) *Moral Problems in Medicine.* Englewood Cliffs, NJ: Prentice-Hall.

Gospel according to Matthew 19, 16ff. New English Bible. Oxford: Oxford University Press and Cambridge University Press.

Macquarrie, J. (ed.) (1967) *A Dictionary of Christian Ethics.* London: SCM Press Ltd.

Niebuhr, R. (1965) cited in Macquarrie, J. (ed.) (1967) *A Dictionary of Christian Ethics.* London: SCM Press Ltd.

Richardson, J. & Webber, I. (1995) *Ethical Issues in Child Health Care.* London: Mosby.

FURTHER READING

Baelz, P. (1977) *Ethics and Belief.* London: Sheldon Press. See in particular Chapter 5, 'Why be Moral?'.

Bayles, M.D. (ed.) (1968) *Contemporary Utilitarianism.* New York: Doubleday.

Gorovitz, S. *et al.* (eds) (1976) *Moral Problems in Medicine.* Englewood Cliffs, NJ: Prentice-Hall.

See in particular Chapter 1, extract from 'Utilitarianism' by John Stuart Mill, and Chapter 2, essays on 'Paternalism'.

Reich, W.T. (1978) *Encyclopedia of Bioethics.* New York: Macmillan and Free Press.

See especially the following articles: 'Ethics: Teleological Theories', Kurt Baier; 'Ethics: Utilitarianism', R.M. Hare; and 'Paternalism', Tom L. Beauchamp.

Seedhouse D. (1988) *Ethics: the Heart of Health Care.* Chichester: J. Wiley & Sons, Ch. 5, The search for morality.

Smart, J.J.C. & Williams, B. (1973) *Utilitarianism – For and Against.* Cambridge: Cambridge University Press.

Thompson, I.E., Melia, K.M. & Boyd, K.M. (1983) *Nursing Ethics.* Edinburgh: Churchill Livingstone.

See in particular Chapter 5 on 'Moral Dilemmas in Nursing Groups of Patients'.

6

Duties, rights, responsibilities

In the preceding chapter the theories discussed judged the rightness or wrongness of an action by its goal. The answer to the question 'Why be moral?' was 'In order to achieve the goal'. The theories discussed in this chapter are not concerned with the goal but more with the act itself. The answers to the question are 'Because we have a *duty* to be moral' or a '*right* to expect morally good behaviour from others' or 'Because we have a *responsibility* toward others'. The act is good in so far as it is in accord with the duty, right or responsibility.

In Chapter 3 we saw that in Judaic law, for example, the physician has a *duty* to treat, and the patient a *duty* to accept treatment, while in Marxist thought there exists the notion that all have a *right* to health care. Professional codes of ethics frequently contain statements which begin, 'The *professional* has a responsibility to ... ' The RCN Code of Professional Conduct discusses the *responsibility* of the nurse 'to patients or clients', 'for professional standards' and 'to colleagues'.

These ideas of duties, rights and responsibilities are frequently applied in all aspects of living. People talk of the duties of parents towards their children, the duties of citizens to report crime, the rights of individuals to education and free speech, and the responsibilities of families for their own members, or of governments towards the citizens of the country.

Before examining theories based on these concepts in more detail it is helpful to try to clarify more fully how they differ from those discussed in Chapter 5. *Teleological*, or goal-based, theories are concerned with the consequences of the act. It is the goal which determines whether the act or rule is morally good or bad.

The theories discussed in this chapter can for the most part be grouped under the heading *deontological* (Greek, deon = duty). The consequences of the act become almost immaterial. What determines if an act is good or bad is whether or not it conforms to our duty or obligation. Thus in judging rightness or wrongness of actions we are examining the opposite ends of the sequence of events. Figure 6.1 illustrates the different emphases between goal-, duty- and rights-based theories.

The goal might be the same in all three situations but that which determines the right act varies. If one begins by defining the goal, one might arrive at a set of duties and rights which are in accord with those of duty- and rights-based theories. It may not necessarily be so, for as we saw in Chapter 5, if the goal is the greatest happiness this does not always lead to a duty to be unselfish. Conversely, if one starts from the point that one has a duty to be unselfish it will almost certainly maximize happiness, at least if happiness is equated with rational pleasure.

From Figure 6.1 it can be seen that in goal-based theories the goal is the primary factor, while any duties or rights derived are secondary. In duty-based theories, where the duty becomes the pri-

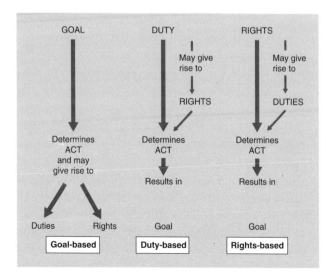

Figure 6.1 The chain of thought and differing emphases of goal-, duty-, and rights-based theories.

mary factor, the goal is of secondary importance. Duties may give rise to rights and vice versa. For example, if I have a *duty* to tell the truth then this gives rise to the idea that you have a *right* to be told the truth. Similarly, if you have a *right* to free speech, then I have a *duty* to allow you that.

DUTY-BASED THEORIES

In utilitarian ethics, the end justifies the means. What duty-based ethics do is place a limit on the means while not necessarily disagreeing with the goodness of the end. For example, if the duty is to preserve life then that is binding. One cannot turn round and say 'but in these particular circumstances the goal (greatest happiness) will be best served by not preserving life'. The duty remains a binding duty even if in acting in accordance with it will do nothing to achieve the goal, or even detract from its achievement.

What can exempt one from acting in accordance with a duty is the obligation to act in accordance with another. It is fairly generally agreed by all duty theorists that to tell the truth is a basic duty. However, one would be justified in not telling the truth in order to comply with the more important duty to preserve life. One would be quite justified in telling a lie in order to prevent the death of another. This is somewhat of a simplification of the position. There might be situations in which truth-telling would take precedence over life preservation. Consider the following situation. Supose you witness a murder and the only penalty for murder in your country is execution. Would you be justified in telling a lie or at least failing to tell the truth in order to save the life of the murderer?

Kant's view of duty was that of the categorical imperative: 'Act only on that maxim that you will to be a universal law.' Kant held that consequences are relatively unimportant but that one has an obligation to act in a particular way because one has a moral duty to do so. Any act performed from a sense of moral duty is morally worthy and, he concluded, can cause no harm. This is fair enough if duties are clearly defined and agreed by all, for then there can be no dispute. The Kantian view is far less definite. It requires a person to exercise his reason and arrive at a logically sound maxim, as tested by the categorical imperative. However, the categorical imperative is insufficiently informative and the individual is left to some extent to decide what his duty is. The duty once defined becomes binding. This could be dangerous if universally applied in health care.

The problem is that this type of duty-based theory totally disregards the desirability of either the means or the consequences. Any action is justified solely on the basis of conformity or non-conformity to the duty. For example, suppose someone considers he has a duty to eliminate a particular disease, say sleeping sickness. This is obviously a quite admirable idea. One way, probably the only way, to eliminate this disease is to eradicate the cause – the tsetse fly. Again, on the face of it an admirable thought. Suppose the only known way of effectively eradicating the tsetse fly is to spray the marshy area in which it thrives with a poison which, in addition to killing the tsetse fly, will be absorbed by fish and kill other animals and birds which eat the fish. Suppose this act sets up a chain of events. The eradication of the tsetse fly renders the area safe for cattle. The cattle move in and consume the lush vegetation, eventually laying the area bare and causing the creation of a barren dust bowl.

A strict interpretation of Kant's theory would be to ignore these and any other consequences, and justify spraying with this particular insecticide because it is in accord with one's duty. Of course, what one has to do is to consider the action in the light of other duties. Does the duty to eliminate sleeping sickness take precedence over the duty to preserve the life of other species, or to maintain the balance of nature?

RIGHTS-BASED THEORIES

'The question of whether health is a right or a privilege is so old and so often asked that it runs the risk of being a cliché' (Fromer, 1981). Before we can begin to discuss rights in health care we need to decide what exactly we mean by a *right*. Generally when we talk of *human rights*, as in the United Nations Declaration, we are talking about natural rights, rights which it is believed exist irrespective of time or place.

Consider these two statements: (a) 'My child has a right to education' and (b) 'I have a right to send my child to the school of my choice.' Statement (a) is talking about a right which many have come to accept as a basic human right, a natural right. Statement (b) is obviously talking about a different type of right. The speaker may have that right if the government has decreed that its citizens should do so but they do not have this right by virtue of being human. Some would argue otherwise. They would say that the right to choose one's child's school is not so much related to the right to education as to another natural right – that is, the right of free choice.

The right of freedom to choose is a particularly thorny one. There must inevitably be some limits placed upon it, if only because one person's right to choose may impinge upon that of someone else. Consider a somewhat simple example. I might claim that I have a right to do whatever I like in my own home. What, then, if I choose to regularly invite some musician friends home to play jazz together into the early hours of the morning? My neighbours would doubtless complain that I and my friends were disturbing their peace and preventing them from sleeping. They might claim that they have a right to a peaceful environment, especially if they had chosen to live in the neighbourhood because it had a reputation for being quiet. They could also claim that they have the right to be able to sleep at nights.

So we begin to see that there are different types of rights. Fromer (1981) distinguishes between two distinct categories of rights: *option* rights and *welfare* rights.

Option rights

The right to choose what I do in my own home is an option right. While in theory one has the right to behave as one pleases, there are limits or boundaries placed upon the extent to which one can exercise such a right. Sometimes the boundaries are clearly defined, as, for example, in defining acceptable modes of dress or undress in certain circumstances. One is free to wear as much or as little as one likes in one's own home, but there are clearly defined boundaries as far as how little one can wear in public. Sometimes the boundaries are less clear cut, as in the case of my claiming a right to play music whenever and however I like in my own home. Sometimes the rights of one individual overlap with those of another and we have to decide which takes priority.

According to Golding (1978), option rights 'should not be taken as implying a general principle to the effect that one has the right to do as one pleases as long as no one else is harmed'. Golding goes on to point out that there may be some things to which one has no rights even though they do no harm to others, and equally there may be some things one has a right to do even if they do harm others.

Option rights are essentially concerned with personal freedom but they are not about total freedom; they do themselves involve an element of control. If I have a right to do as I please within the boundary of allowed behavior, what Fromer describes as my 'sphere of sovereignty', then you have no right to prevent me exercising mine. If my actions go beyond the defined boundary or sphere then you have a right to stop me. Indeed, it is option rights which are the basis of most, if not all, suits in civil courts. A sues B because B has either prevented A from exerting his rights, or because A has been unable to stop B when B has gone outside his sphere.

Welfare rights

Welfare rights are rights granted by law. Thus in the United Kingdom, for example, one can claim a right to expect a certain standard of safety in building construction, a right to clean air, a right to a secret vote in parliamentary elections and so on. Conflict arises when individuals lay claim to rights not granted in law but which are an integral part of their own moral code. If sufficient numbers lay claim to a right that does not exist, then it might be that they can bring pressure to bear to bring about a change in the law and the creation of a new welfare right. Welfare rights are about benefits or legal entitlement. I have the right to expect something or to receive something, whereas, as we have seen, option rights are concerned with personal freedom.

Implication of rights-based theories

The notions of freedom and possession of rights are clearly intertwined. You cannot have freedom without having rights. Although the reverse is not necessarily true, it is possible to accept the idea that people have certain rights without allowing them total freedom. A society might concur with the idea that citizens have a right to education without allowing them the freedom of choosing whether to exercise that right. It might also be held that they have a duty to be educated. Even in a totalitarian state the citizens may have some welfare rights but have little personal freedom. Nevertheless, there is a positive relationship between freedom and rights, as Figure 6.2 illustrates.

Now, if possession of rights implies freedom, it follows that one has the freedom to choose whether or not to exert one's rights. For example, I may have a right, a welfare right, to health care but choose not to request care when I am ill. I have the right not to exercise my right. On the face of it that may appear to pose little difficulty. If I choose not to have my illness treated that is my affair; I might be accused of behaving foolishly but not immorally – not, that is, unless my not exercising my right prevents others from exercising theirs. It could be argued that if my illness were infectious, in choosing to not have it treated I would be denying those around me the right to live in a healthy environment.

On the other hand, if another of my rights, an option right, is freedom of control over my own body, then I have every right to decide what I will allow others to do to it. I have the right to decide whether I want it washed, prodded and examined, massaged, X- rayed, perforated by needles and any of the other things that health workers might want to do to it. It follows that if my decision is to be based on reason rather than emotion I also have

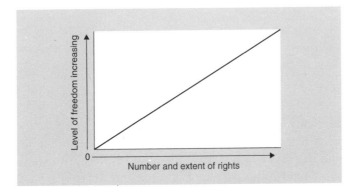

Figure 6.2 Relationship between level of freedom and the number and extent of rights.

the right to be given sufficient information on which to base my decision. And just as I have the right not to exercise my rights I also have the right to do so.

We begin to see that rights, whatever their source or nature, can not exist in isolation. If everyone based all their actions on their rights and their freedom to choose whether or not to exercise their rights with no concern for others, then chaos would ensue. There is a need for some kind of control. The control may be self-regulating, as is the case quite often with option rights, or it may be a legal one or a moral one.

Let us assume that a government accepts that every child has a right to a free education. The government automatically imposes upon itself the duty to provide the opportunity for every child to receive a free education. There is nothing to stop a child's parents from paying for an education and not exercising the right to a free education. Nor is there anything to stop them from not exerting their right in another way, by opting out altogether. Obviously if everyone chose the latter course the result would be disastrous and, even if a few chose it, it would be less than desirable. The government can of course manipulate the situation by legislating that parents must ensure that their children receive an education and can insist that the free State education will be the only provision.

In this situation the government has defined (a) a right and (b) a duty. The right is a welfare right and the control is a legal duty. However, not all duties are defined by law. The government, in recognizing the right of its citizens to a free education, automatically becomes duty-bound to provide the means. This is frequently the consequence of accepting rights. Some would argue that it was always the consequence.

Let us return to the question of rights in health care. Earlier I referred to my right as a patient to choose not to seek health care. The extent to which I can exert that right is, I suggested, controlled by the rights of others. It could also be argued that it is controlled by my duty towards others: that is, a moral duty not to act deliberately in any way which will harm others. Obviously, if I choose to exert my right to health care, it has implications in that someone has a duty to provide it. The implications of my exerting my rights *in* rather than *to* health care are more far-reaching.

'The granting of rights automatically implies corresponding duties and responsibilities; one cannot exist without the other' (Former, 1981). If a patient chooses to exercise his or her right to have his or her treatment explained to him, then someone has an obligation to give him or her the information. The question of information-giving will be explored more fully in Chapter 11. Here we merely establish the consequences of rights-based theories in health care. So let us turn our attention to some other rights. 'I have the right to be free from pain' (*The Dying Person's Bill of Rights*). If a patient has the right to be free from pain, then health carers have a duty to keep the patient free from pain. The question which immediately arises is whether it is always possible to keep the patient free from pain. What if no known analgesics are effective or if the only effective ones are unavailable? What if the only way to relieve the pain is to give a lethal dose of a drug?

If a patient has the right to choose whether or not to undergo a particular treatment and chooses not to do so, then the carer has a duty to allow the patient that choice. If that choice in no way endangers the patient's life or if it will have little or no effect on the course of their illness or recovery, then there is no real problem. For example, if a patient refuses a bed-bath then the nurse would have little difficulty in complying with that decision. What if the patient refuses to undergo life-saving surgery or to have a life-sustaining drug such as insulin?

The answers to questions such as those posed at the ends of the last two paragraphs are two-fold. Firstly, it might be argued that the patient has a duty to promote their own health and therefore to undergo appropriate treatment to that end. Secondly, the health professionals might argue that they have a duty which supersedes all others and that is the duty to preserve life. They therefore have no right to refuse to carry out treatment or to refuse not to carry out treatment which will contradict that duty. They could argue that the patient cannot refuse the treatment or that if he or she does, then their duty is to override the patient's wishes.

The duty to promote one's own health could be said to be derived from a right to health, if such a right exists. A right to health is not the same as a right to health care. The latter is becoming a generally accepted right, while the former has not been established and is to some extent an unrealistic expectation. It is not as yet possible to prevent or cure all illness. Therefore, the duty to promote one's own health is not derived from a right and is a basic duty.

To rely solely on rights-based theories in making ethical decisions would result in frequent conflict and almost certain chaos. Certainly, in the practice of health care it frequently becomes necessary to appeal to some other basis for making decisions. Rights-based theories do not provide a sufficiently structured framework to encompass the whole gamut of moral decisions. Nevertheless, the notion of rights, and of natural rights in particular, has brought a vital dimension to the ethics of health care which traditionally have relied heavily on the notion of duties. It is the increasing acceptance of the concept of a right to health care that has brought increased motivation to remove inequalities in health care both within and between nations.

RESPONSIBILITIES

'The fundamental responsibility of the nurse is four-fold: to promote health, to prevent illness, to restore health and to alleviate suffering' (International Council of Nurses, 1973). As already noted, codes of professional ethics frequently contain statements about the responsibilities of the members of the profession. Benjamin and Curtis (1992) describe such statements as that quoted from the ICN Code as *statements of creed*, as opposed to *commandments*, for such statements are not so much directives to behave in a particular way as statements of belief; they are saying something about what the profession believes to be the nature of, in this case, nursing.

'As creeds, codes of nursing ethics provide a valuable reminder of the special responsibilities incumbent upon those who tend the sick' (Benjamin and Curtis, 1992). Patients or clients are vulnerable, particularly if they are sick or handicapped. They may be very dependent upon the nurse, not just to provide them with their physical needs but to protect them from abuse or deceit. If as a result of illness the patient suffers a loss of hearing, sight or reasoning power, then they may be frightened and very vulnerable. They may have difficulty in understanding the explanation of their treatment. The patient may, albeit temporarily, be unable to make a rational and objective choice between alternatives even if they are offered one. The nurse has a responsibility to help the patient understand more fully the information presented. However, nurses should not use their advantaged position afforded by knowledge and skills to persuade the patient to make one choice rather than another. As Francis Bacon said, 'knowledge is power'. It is a criticism frequently levied at professions that they keep their body of knowledge to themselves in order to maintain, even increase, their power in society.

'The primary responsibility of nurses is to protect and enhance the well-being and dignity of each individual in their care' (RCN Code, 1976). Patients are vulnerable not only because of physical or mental impairment. Sadly, nurses and other health professionals frequently increase the patient's vulnerability by reducing, rather than enhancing, their dignity. The patient is placed in unfamiliar surroundings – namely, a hospital or clinic. They are required to dress in night clothes even though it is daytime and even if they are able to be up and about. Most of the conversations between professional and patient take place while the patient is lying on a bed or couch. The professional wears at best normal daytime clothes or at worst a uniform. All these factors only serve to increase the patient's vulnerability. It is almost impossible to converse on equal terms with someone else when you are wearing night clothes and they are wearing a uniform. It makes it difficult for the patient to ask for explanations of their illness and its treatment. It makes it easy for the professional to tell patients what is 'best' for them, to take control of them.

Nurses have responsibilities not only to their patients but to the profession and to society as a whole. 'As a registered nurse, midwife or health visitor, you … in the exercise of your professional accountability, must: assist professional colleagues, in the context of your own knowledge, experience and sphere of responsibility, to develop their professional competence' (UKCC, 1992).

Nurses have a responsibility not just to ensure that their own knowledge and skills are constantly being improved but also to contribute to the development of knowledge and skills within the profession as a whole. This means that nurses cannot view the job solely in terms of their direct interactions with patients but have to have regard for the needs of colleagues. The full clause (Clause 14) of the UKCC Code of Conduct expands the responsibility of the nurse to include not only his or her professional peers and subordinates but also others in the care team, including informal carers.

The nurse's responsibility to the profession is wider even than that. Item eight of the American Nurses' Association (ANA) *Code for Nurses* states that 'The nurse participates in the profession's efforts to implement and improve standards of nursing'. This suggests that each individual nurse has a responsibility not just for local standards of care but for contributing to the enhancement of the standards of the profession as a whole. It seems to me implicit in this statement that nurses have a responsibility to be actively involved in whatever machinery exists for promoting standards of care. This would include active membership of professional associations, full involvement in the organizational structure in which they work, and being engaged in research. It also would seem to imply that their responsibility does not cease with the end of the working day.

The pursuit of enhancing standards of care may well bring an individual nurse into conflict with colleagues. It has frequently been said that a nurse's responsibility to the profession, or that of any professional to his or her profession, means protecting the profession from criticism. 'Always support your colleagues in public.' Professions, and nursing is no exception, have a tradition of *closing* ranks when faced with criticism from outside. Professions should welcome such criticism, even invite it, and members of the profession should, if they feel the criticism to be justified, add their support to it. If nurses are prepared to question their practices and to explore alternatives, then one of the main aims of the profession – namely, to improve standards of care – will be better served.

It is not only its own actions and decisions which a profession should question but also those of others inasmuch as they affect its sphere of concern. Thus nurses have a responsibility to society to concern themselves with the decisions and actions of other health-care professions, and also those of politicians when they affect the health status and care of the community. If a government cuts the amount it spends on health care or refuses to initiate legislation to decrease environmental pollution, then nurses, singly and collectively, ought to have something to say. Indeed, they have a responsibility to society to say it.

SUMMARY

In this chapter we have considered alternative answers to the question 'Why be moral?' The three answers examined have been (a) because I have a duty ..., (b) because he has a right to ... and (c) because I have a responsibility. Duties and rights may be natural or basic – that is, existing as part of the natural order of things. Alternatively, they may be contrived – that is, defined by man or by a particular society. Such duties and rights can, of course, be as easily abolished as they are created. Both duty- and rights-based theories have made major impacts on the ethics of health care but, as we have seen, neither on their own provides sufficient framework for all decision-making.

Whereas duties and rights are an integral part of societal or cultural ethics, responsibilities, as discussed here, are part of professional ethics. Because they are nurses, nurses have certain moral responsibilities that are not shared by other members of society.

REFERENCES

American Nurses' Association (1976) *Code for Nurses.*

Benjamin, M. & Curtis, J. (1992) *Ethics in Nursing,* 3rd edn. New York: Oxford University Press.

Fromer, M.J. (1981) *Ethical Issues in Health Care.* St Louis: C.V. Mosby.

Golding, M.P. (1978) cited in Fromer, M.J. (1981) *Ethical Issues in Health Care.* St Louis: C.V. Mosby.

International Council of Nurses. (1973) *Code for Nurses: Ethical Concepts Applied to Nursing.* Geneva: ICN.

Royal College of Nursing (1976) *RCN Code of Professional Conduct – a Discussion Document.* London: RCN.

UKCC (United Kingdom Central Council for Nursing, Midwifery and Health Visiting) (1992) *Code of Professional Conduct for the Nurse, Midwife and Health Visitor,* 3rd edn. London: UKCC.

The Dying Person's Bill of Rights, created at a workshop on 'The Terminally Ill Patient and the Helping Person', in Lansing, Michigan, USA.

FURTHER READING

Bandman, B. & Bandman, E.L. (1978) *Bioethics and Human Rights.* Boston: Little, Brown.

Fromer, M.J. (1981) *Ethical Issues in Health Care.* St Louis: C.V. Mosby.

See in particular Chapter 1 on 'Professional Accountability' and Chapter 2 on 'Justice and Allocation in Health Care'.

Reich, W.T. (1978) *Encyclopedia of Bioethics.* New York: Macmillan and Free Press.

See especially the following articles: 'Ethics: Deontological Theories', Kurt Baier; 'Health Care: Right to Health Care Services', Albert R. Jonsen; and 'Rights: Rights in Bioethics', Ruth Macklin.

Richardson, J. & Webber, I. (1995) *Ethical Issues in Child Health Care.* London: Mosby.

See in particular Chapter 4 on 'Rights'.

Ross, D. (1969) *Kant's Ethical Theory.* Oxford: Oxford University Press.

Thompson, I.E., Melia, K.M. & Boyd, K.M. (1988) *Nursing Ethics,* 2nd edn. Edinburgh: Churchill Livingstone.

See in particular Chapter 3 on 'Responsibility and Accountability'.

7

Death and dying

This chapter explores a number of ethical issues related to the end of life. It begins with an exploration of the arguments for and against euthanasia; it then goes on to discuss more specific issues which draw into focus some of the differences between medical and nursing ethics discussed in Chapter 1, in particular decisions to discontinue or withdraw treatment. The case of Tony Bland is used as a basis for this discussion. The relationship between law and ethics is discussed both in the light of the Tony Bland case and *advanced directives*.

EUTHANASIA

Euthanasia has for many years been a controversial issue both within and outside the health professions, and there exist several misconceptions as to what it actually means. Therefore, before examining the various arguments surrounding the act of euthanasia it is necessary to define what is meant by it.

The word *euthanasia* is derived from the Greek words *eu* and *thanatos*, and literally means a gentle or easy death. As such it is probably every person's hope, for most would not wish for a sudden death nor would they wish for a lingering one. A dying person expects their doctor to be able to make death, when it comes, as easy and pain-free as possible, and today this is possible in the majority of cases when it is known that death is impending. To this literal meaning of *euthanasia* there can be no moral objection. However, in modern usage, the word *euthanasia* has taken on a very different meaning. It has come to mean *the painless killing of men and women to end their sufferings*, and it is often referred to as *mercy killing*.

It is euthanasia in this latter sense with which we are concerned here: the deliberate ending of life, either voluntarily or involuntarily, on the grounds of humanity, as distinct from murder, which does not generally have the interests of the victim or society at heart. However, this definition requires some further clarification and it is necessary to define those acts which can or cannot be said to be included within it.

Take for example the case considered in Chapter 2. In that situation the doctor was faced with the decision to give or not to give analgesics, the dosage of which, required to relieve the patient's pain, would inevitably hasten death. The question we now ask is 'Can this be called euthanasia?' The answer is '*Yes*' in the literal sense, for what the doctor is doing is relieving the patient of pain and thus making the process of dying easier, but '*No*' in the sense under discussion here, because the doctor is not deliberately setting out to end the patient's life.

Another act which is often referred to as mercy killing is the decision of a doctor not to resuscitate a patient but allow them to die quickly and naturally. The law, at least in the United Kingdom, does not call this killing, again because the doctor is not deliberately killing the patient. Not to throw a lifebelt to a drowning man would be morally indefensible in the view of the majority of people; whereas not to resuscitate a dying man when to do so would only stave off the moment of death or result in a prolonged and unpleasant death, or a cabbage-like existence, can be morally defended. It can be argued that preserving physical existence when there is no mental or spiritual existence is not preserving human life.

Acts such as these are often referred to as *passive euthanasia*, and it is argued that such acts can be morally justified. My concern here is less with passive euthanasia and more with active euthanasia. The two ideas can be clearly differentiated. Passive euthanasia can be defined as '*cooperating with the patient's dying*' (Nelson, 1973), and active euthanasia has been defined as '*those techniques and procedures deliberately intended to interrupt the patient's ability to sustain life, to legalise which an Act of Parliament would be necessary*' (Nelson, 1973).

The case for euthanasia

In defence of active or positive euthanasia, Fletcher (1973) argues that 'It is harder morally to justify letting somebody die a slow and ugly death, dehumanised, than it is to justify helping him to escape from such misery'. Fletcher argues that what we should be concerned with is the preservation of humanness and personal integrity above biological life and function. 'The traditional ethics based on the sanctity of life ... must give way to a code of ethics of the quality of life.'

People are more than biological beings; they are rational beings. When the rational element is lost, it is argued, then what is left is less than human. There is therefore no obligation to preserve the life of an individual who has lost cerebral capacity and is no longer able to rationalize or express emotion but is still capable of physiological functioning (an argument which is further discussed later in this chapter). Thus, it is argued that it is justifiable to end the life of a person whose ability to reason has been lost due to trauma or disease, or who due to congenital defects will never acquire that ability. Persons who are incapable of rationalizing are by definition not *human*. Furthermore, since such persons are incapable of rational thought, they would be unable to make a decision for themselves as to whether they should live or die. Someone else would make the decision for them and would, according to this school of thought, be morally justified in so doing.

Modern medicine has given us considerable control over the birth process, and it has also opened up new possibilities for resuscitation and prolonging life. We are therefore forced to make decisions about death as much as about birth. Those in favour of euthanasia would argue that there must be the same quality control in the terminating of life as in its initiating. 'It is ridiculous to give ethical approval to the terminating of subhuman life *in utero*, as we do in therapeutic abortions for reasons of mercy and compassion, but refuse to approve positively ending life *in extremis*' (Fletcher, 1973).

Earlier, I argued that there is a very clear distinction between passive and active euthanasia. Many supporters of euthanasia would disagree with such a view. They argue that there is no such moral distinction between the two acts, between letting die and killing. Since the former is accepted in certain circumstances (for example, a patient on a life-support system who stands no chance of recovery), then the latter must also be acceptable.

*There seems in fact to be no general difference between the obliga-
tion not to cause harm and the obligation to prevent harm, and no
general difference between the obligation to refrain from killing
others and the obligation not to let others die. Hence there is little
if any basis for thinking that active and passive euthanasia differ
in some morally significant way.*

(Montague, 1978)

Therefore, it follows that since passive euthanasia is practised and
morally defensible, there is no reason to disallow active euthanasia.
The argument of course works both ways; if there is no moral difference between the two, then neither should be allowed.

As was discussed in Chapter 2, one way of deciding whether an
act is right or wrong is to consider the extent to which the end
result serves humane values. Proponents of an end-justifies-the-
means ethic would argue that in some circumstances the end
(death) does justify the act of deliberately bringing it about. No life,
it is argued, is better than dehumanized life. As has already been
noted, Clause 1 of the Code of Conduct is paramount to the
exercising of professional accountability. The case for euthanasia
depends upon an understanding of the terms *well-being* and
interests of the patient. It can be argued that there are instances in
which death may be in the *patient's interests,* and that to maintain
life may in fact not promote their *well-being* inasmuch as the
patient is forced to continue a life the quality of which is extremely
poor.

One further argument used by some advocates of euthanasia
concerns the rights of the individual. Since 1961 it has ceased to be
illegal (in the United Kingdom) to take one's own life. Therefore, it
is argued, in law at least, that one has the right to end one's life. It
follows then that if one desires to bring one's life to an end, but
does not have the means or ability to do so, one has the right to
ask another to assist one in the act. The basis of the argument is
that everyone is entitled to live their life in accordance with their
own value system, and that no one has the right to impose a set of
values upon another. This right to live according to one's own values extends to death, a view supported to some extent by Clause 6
of the Code of Conduct. I purposely say 'to some extent' because

this clause is not as prescriptive as several of the others. It merely requires the nurse 'to *take account* of the customs' (my emphasis). Clearly, it is envisaged that there might be situations in which allowing patients a right to exercise their customs, values or spiritual beliefs may be harmful to them or others.

One of the weaknesses of the argument that patients should be allowed to demand euthanasia because it accords with their beliefs and values, is that society would be requiring doctors and nurses to relinquish the very rights that would be given to patients. If euthanasia were to become lawful, presumably nurses would be able to invoke Clause 7 of the Code of Conduct. However, this clause, like Clause 6, is open to misinterpretation. The nurse is required to '*make known* ... any conscientious objection' (again my emphasis). There is no implied requirement that the nurse be allowed to exercise that conscientious objection. It is to be hoped, therefore, that were a Euthanasia Bill ever to be enacted, it would contain a clause, as does the Abortion Act, affording health professionals the right to refuse to participate in the procedure.

One of the vital differences between man and the animals is that man has the *capacity for death by choice*, and thus the use of this option puts man on an entirely different plane from other animals, which we may decide simply to put to death when the appropriate time occurs. If a person exercises their *right* of death by choice, they can also donate a vital organ and know that the necessary operation can be arranged in advance and the time of death established without any doubt or difficulty. So to choose the moment of our death when suffering from an incurable disease seems both merciful to the individual, and also may be of benefit to others. The *right to die* has become something of a basic principle in the campaign to legalize euthanasia. It is the principle behind the request of many relatives that a life support machine be switched off when the patient has been, for all human purposes, apparently dead for some time, and that of Tony Bland's parents for all active treatment to be ended when he was in a *persistent vegetative state* (we will return to this latter case later in this chapter). And, it is the principle behind the desire to allow sufferers from an incurable disease to say when the time has come to welcome death.

The case against euthanasia

Fletcher claims that it is harder to justify letting someone die slowly than it is to give that person a lethal injection. His argument is based upon a *personalistic* or *humanistic* code of ethics. He argues that life in itself is not important, that it is rationality and personality that make a person human. While one might agree with him that persons are composed of many facets – personal and physical, spiritual and corporeal – one might well argue that he over-emphasizes the personality and soul to the detriment of the physical. 'To say that existence is not sufficient reason for an individual to be recognised as human is to almost totally exclude the physical dimension of man' (Weber, 1973). The body, although it may be a temporary thing, unlike the spirit which may live on after death, is still an essential element of humanness. It is the embodied person with which doctors and nurses are concerned; it is the physical being which is presented to them for their care and treatment. To violate the physical body is to violate the human person as much as violating the personality.

When one thinks of the person as a combination of the spiritual and the physical, it is less difficult to differentiate between letting a terminally ill patient die and directly ending the life of a patient. 'The point is, of course, that killing a patient removes his chances of recovery in a way that allowing him to die does not' (Montague, 1978). There is a defensible and valid distinction between killing and letting die. Those who would want to prolong life at all costs fall into the trap of placing too much emphasis on the physical, while those who argue in favour of euthanasia frequently place too much emphasis on the personality. It is the needs of the total person that we have to consider.

The needs of the terminally ill patient may be best served not by attempting to extend their life, but by concentrating on their needs as a dying person. 'Respect for a dying person may demand that we stop the art of healing so that we can help the patient practise what medieval man called *ars morendi,* the art of dying' (Weber, 1973). Active euthanasia is something very different. It is not an attempt to meet the needs of a dying person, but a direct ending of their life, and as such is a violation of the person. Death becomes the result, not of disease, but of the act of a human agent. The difference is a very important one which should not be ignored, for as Weber has it:

> There is an enormous difference between not fighting death and actively putting an end to life. The former is fully compatible with respect for human life. The latter, while done with the best intentions, is logically part of the view that human life itself is not enough to warrant our respect.

The quality-of-life ethic, when used to support active euthanasia, is in danger of self-contradiction. Those who support such a view are in effect saying that, in order to improve the quality of life, it may be necessary to destroy it. Furthermore, the case for euthanasia would extend beyond that of the terminally ill patient who has become dehumanized and would, for example, justify the killing of babies born with such disorders as Down's syndrome, whereas the sanctity-of-life approach argues that the quality of all life suffers if life itself becomes violable. Unless every human life is considered of value because of its very existence, then the quality of life itself is devalued.

To followers of all the major world religions, life is sacred, and therefore all ethical decisions must be grounded in a reverence for life. In some religions, notably Judaism, Christianity and Islam, there is the added dimension of belief in a God who is creator. Life is given, and therefore can only be taken, by God or Allah. The problem is, as was discussed in Chapter 3, that the major religious writings such as the Bible and the Koran do not contain mention of many of the specific moral issues such as euthanasia which we face today. What they do contain are sets of moral or ethical principles. The principle that concerns us here is *Thou shalt not kill*, and for many that is the end of the argument. 'Thou shalt not kill therefore euthanasia is wrong.' However, as we saw in Chapter 3, almost all religious traditions allow killing in certain circumstances. Some Christians, for example, would argue that in certain situations, deliberately to end the life of a patient would be justified on the grounds that it was the more loving thing to do, and that the principle to show love is the predominant one. Other religious traditions, such as Hinduism and Buddhism, take a stronger view and argue that killing can never be justified.

The second principle on which Christians and others base their argument is the law of nature. 'Some theologians have argued that God's will is reflected in nature and that to act against nature is to act against the will of God. To terminate life, and not let nature take its course, is to act immorally' (Rayner, 1976). Similarly, Muslims would argue that everything is in the hands of Allah and that what Allah wills will happen. Thus intervention is futile. The obvious flaw in the argument, as Rayner points out, is that it goes too far. Most, if not all, medical practice is an interference with the course of nature. Were it not for the advances in antenatal care, preventive medicine and antibiotics, many of the now incurably ill would not have survived to contract their present disease. Therefore, since medical interference is partly responsible for the problem, it would seem ridiculous not to interfere with nature in order to solve the problem. The argument should not be about whether to interfere with nature, but about the form that interference should take.

With euthanasia, as with many other ethical issues, to argue for it on the basis that the end justifies the means is to place emphasis on the reason for acting rather than on the action itself. 'By concentrating almost exclusively on the proposed end of serving human happiness and well-being, ethicists of the end-justifies-the-means variety seem to forget sometimes that the means chosen can deny the ends desired' (Weber, 1973). Fletcher argues that by ending a person's life, one can be providing for his well-being. The question is, if he is losing his life, his *being*, can this really be said to serve his *well-being*? It is hard to see how a person's quality of life can be improved by the ending of it.

That those who would support the introduction of legalized active euthanasia are guided by humane and loving motives cannot be denied. Their concern is for the well-being of the individual and the preservation of human dignity. However, while it must be admitted that some patients suffering from incurable diseases do suffer extreme pain, and some do die in agony of body and mind, the question remains whether euthanasia is the best answer to the problem. In recent years, medical science has made great strides not only in heroic life-saving surgery and technological medicine, but also in the less dramatic field of pain control. The work of those involved in the hospice movement has shown that it is possible to control both physical and mental pain even in the terminal stages of malignant disease. While a lot still remains to be done, this surely is the direction in which medicine and nursing should move, for this is working towards a positive solution to the problem, whereas euthanasia is a negative and defeatist solution. It has been shown that death with dignity is possible without resorting to a deliberate hastening of the process.

The *right-to-die* argument is claimed by many to be unfounded, for we have a right to die inasmuch as it is an inevitable condition of life itself. We do not have a right to choose when or how we will die any more than we can choose when we will be born. True, the former is a technical possibility while the latter is obviously impossible, but ability to do something is not in itself a right to do it. Nor can the right to *die* be compared to the right to *life* of the *Declaration of Human Rights*, for closely bound up in that right to life is the notion that no one has the right to take the life of another. Any form of involuntary euthanasia is thus most definitely not justifiable. Any attempt to choose the moment of our death is really a claim to a right to suicide, and although suicide is not illegal, it is not therefore automatically morally defensible. Nor should a right to die be confused with the genuine, common-sense conclusion frequently reached by doctors that nature take its course and a patient, whose life is being artificially prolonged or who is already dead in effect, should be allowed to die. In fact, in such cases as will be discussed later, to prolong life unnecessarily could be said to be interfering with a person's right to die in a more acceptable sense of the phrase – the inevitability of death.

NOT PROLONGING LIFE

So far in this chapter we have been concerned with the ethics of decisions to end life. We now turn our attention to decisions about whether or not to prolong life. Two areas will be explored. First the decision not to resuscitate, and second, decisions to commence or cease life-prolonging treatment.

Do not resuscitate orders

Do not resuscitate orders raise several ethical questions, not least for the nurse. Firstly, there is the question of who should decide. Frequently it is the doctor who decides and makes that decision on a judgement of the patient's expected quality of life – something which in many cases can only be guessed at and not known for certain. Bandman and Bandman (1990) argue that it should not be the health professional who decides but the patient: 'playing God by deciding who has the required quality of life and who therefore lives or dies also reveals a serious moral pitfall of arbitrarily abridging the equal rights of individuals to decide whether to live or die.'

However, allowing the patient to decide does not totally relieve nurses of moral conflicts. In some ways the UKCC Code of Conduct does not help to resolve these conflicts, but serves to emphasize them. Clauses 1 and 2 require the nurse to act always in such a way as to 'promote and safeguard the interests and well-being of patients' and 'to ensure that no act or omission on his/her part ... is detrimental to the condition or safety of patients/clients'. Not to resuscitate in some instances, even if in accordance with the patient's wishes, could be judged to be not promoting their well-being and to be detrimental to them. On the other hand, Clause 6 requires the nurse 'To take account of the customs, values and spiritual beliefs of patients/clients'. The nurse who does not comply with a patient's request not to be resuscitated could be said to be violating this clause. The question for the nurse to resolve is which clause takes precedence. It would seem evident from the way in which the Code is set out and from subsequent UKCC advisory documents, such as 'Exercising Accountability' (1989) that Clause 1 is paramount.

A further problem which nurses face is of a more practical nature. How do they know whether to resuscitate or not? According to Aarons and Beeching (1991), in many British hospitals clear guidelines do not exist, and of equal concern is that 'Elective decisions not to resuscitate are not effectively communicated to nurses'. They conclude by saying, 'We advocate more discussion of patients' suitability for resuscitation between doctors, nurses, patients and patients' relatives.'

Withdrawal of life-sustaining treatment

'How ought we to treat and care for patients who are dying? There are usually many things we can do but it is sometimes questionable whether they are all worth doing.' (Campbell, 1995). There are, it seems, two issues that should be explored when treating those who are nearing death. The first is whether or not to initiate life-prolonging treatment when there is no possibility of cure and the second is when to cease treating. It is with the second of these issues that we are most concerned here. However, in many instances the reason that decisions have to be made about if and when to cease treating is because an earlier decision has been taken to commence treatment in the first place. The second issue therefore raises questions about the first.

Decisions to commence life-prolonging treatment

Let us consider first a situation in which the patient requests life-prolonging treatment. Taken at face value, and assuming that the request is based on a full knowledge of the situation and made by a person who is judged to be capable of rational thought, this would seem to pose no dilemma. However, it is seldom that simple. Two ethical principles are relevant to the discussion – the principle of justice, and the principle of autonomy.

First the health professional needs to consider the individual case in the light of available resources. Resources in health care are limited and there may not be sufficient resources to meet every request for life-prolonging treatment. The question is how do we decide? In this, as in other areas of health care where decisions have to be made as to who gets what, it is helpful to have agreed criteria. If there are clearly laid down criteria for determining whether a person should be eligible for a particular treatment, then it relieves the professional from having to make a choice between competing claims. Each case is judged on its own merits. Age might be a criterion. It was applied, for example, in the early days of renal dialysis. Quality of life years (QALYs) might be another criterion. The question of justice in health care, and that of QALYs are more fully discussed in Chapter 13.

Whether or not resources are available, and especially if they are, there is also a need to consider the principle of autonomy. The Stanley Report (1992) suggests that the individual's autonomous decision might be overridden on three grounds. First, if the health team consider the treatment will be futile in the sense of not achieving the desired physiological change; second, if the treatment involves pain disproportionate to the hoped for benefit; third, if a member of the health care team has a conscientious objection to the required treatment. Singleton and McLaren (1995) argue that none of these are adequate reasons for overriding an individual's autonomous decision:

> *The first two points appear to throw doubt on whether the original decision was really autonomous ... If the treatment will definitely not achieve the desired physiological change, then it would be irrational to request it ... Benefits and pains are a matter for the individual to assess and will be reflected in the individual's autonomous decision. To allow for the overriding of an individual's autonomy on these grounds is to open the way for paternalistic infringements of individuals' autonomy.*

The answer to the third point raised in the Stanley Report would be simply to refer the case to another health professional.

So far we have been concerned with requests to commence life-prolonging treatment made by the patient. Many patients about whom such decisions have to be made are not themselves capable of being involved in the decision-making process, those for example in a *persistent vegetative state* (PVS), and so we move now to consider the issue from a professional decision-making viewpoint. The Stanley Report (1992) asserts that such patients have no self-regarding interests, and goes on to state that it follows that there are no patient-based reasons for continuing life-sustaining treatment. However, one cannot totally disregard the patient when making the decision.

...a knowledge of the individual's previous values and ideals is relevant when considering the continuation [or commencement] of life-sustaining treatments.' (Singleton and McLaren, 1995). Knowledge of their values and ideals may be obtained from their relatives, if there are any, or may already be known to the health professional through previous involvement in their care. The point is that although at this point in time the patient has no actual interests since they have lost all powers of cognition and sentience, they were previously an autonomous agent. And, if their previous wishes and or beliefs are known, these should be taken into account when making the decision. The interests and wishes of the family also need to be taken into consideration. However, at the end of the day it is a decision for the health care team and their values also play a part. And, as noted in the earlier discussion, the availability of resources is a factor to be considered. The overriding consideration has to be what course of action is in the patient's best interests – will be treatment enhance not only the length but also the quality of their life? – coupled with an informed judgement about their wishes had they still a decision-making capacity.

Discontinuation of treatment

There are cases in which, in retrospect, it would seem better not to have commenced treatment other than that aimed at symptom control. Campbell (1995) cites the example of a 68-year-old man dying of an inoperable cancer of the stomach. In this case the patient was first treated by palliative removal of part of the stomach. Shortly following the first operation the patient developed a pulmonary embolism which was removed by an operation. This in turn was followed by a myocardial infarction and the patient was resuscitated. On four further occasions the patient's heart stopped and was artificially restarted. The result was that the patient suffered brain damage and survived a few more weeks in severe pain.

The decision had been made to attempt every possible procedure to prolong the patient's life. While these attempts resulted in prolonging the patient's life, they also resulted in causing the patient increased suffering, both directly as a result of the procedures and as a result of the spread of the cancer. The quality of the patient's life and death was greatly reduced, when, had the decision been made to cease active intervention at an earlier stage, following the first operation or treatment of the embolus, he might have enjoyed a shorter life of better quality and a more dignified death.

The problem is that once a decision has been taken to initiate treatment it becomes increasingly difficult to make the decision to cease treating. However, there is much support for the view that life-prolonging treatment might rightly be withdrawn from a patient who is dying:

The cessation of the employment of extraordinary means to prolong the life of the body when there is irrefutable evidence that biological death is imminent is the decision of the patient and/or his immediate family.

(American Medical Association, 1974)

This view is also supported by the British Medical Association (1981).

However, as in the decision to commence treatment, the patient may not be capable of making a contribution. Nevertheless, the decision should still not rest with one health professional:

In the case of the PVS patient, the determination of irreversibility can only be made by doctors ... the determination of continued treatment as futile and thus optional, should be a shared judgement.

(Mitchell *et al.*, 1993)

That judgement should involve not just the doctor and the patient's relatives/significant others but also other members of the health care team. It is often the nurse who is most closely involved with the patient and their family, and who more often, therefore, has a fuller understanding of their wishes and values. The decision to cease life-sustaining treatment is not a purely clinical one, it is equally an ethical one, and 'Expertise in clinical diagnosis does not automatically confer expertise in ethical decision-making.' (Singleton and McLaren, 1995).

The issues surrounding the decision to cease life-prolonging treatment were drawn into the public domain as a result of the case of Tony Bland. Tony Bland was a victim of the Hillsborough football stadium disaster (April 1989). His injuries rendered him comatose and he remained in a persistent vegetative state until 1993 when his parents applied through the courts to have active treatment discontinued. What is significant in this case is the precise nature of the treatment concerned. It was not treatment which one would normally consider falling under the umbrella of *extraordinary means*. It was the withdrawal of artificial nutrition and hydration and for antibiotics not to be given for which the parents requested permission.

The ruling of the courts was equally significant. First, they held that artificial nutrition and hydration constituted treatment, and second, that because the patient would not recover, the treatment was of no benefit to him, and that withdrawing it would take the form of legal omission rather than commission. The medical team, in the view of the courts, had no duty to continue treating Tony Bland.

The principle here was that '*caring* for a patient (in cases where care was not possible and recovery was extremely unlikely) did not require medical interventions which were of no benefit to the patient.' (Campbell, 1995). That they were of no benefit in terms of effecting a cure is not debatable; however, it could be argued that they were of benefit in terms of maintaining the patient's physical well-being. Furthermore, as Campbell (1995) points out, the treatment was certainly not a *disbenefit* and did the patient no harm.

However, patients, especially in situations such as this, cannot be considered in isolation. Given Bland's condition, action or inaction was not likely to affect him in any sense in which he would be consciously aware of the effects. The decisions and actions did have an effect on his family. They were the ones who had consciously suffered as a result of effects of the injuries suffered by Tony. The decision to cease treatment was a benefit to them. For them it brought about an end of two years of anxiously watching their son in a distressing condition, and enabled them at last to fully mourn their loss. This is a significant benefit, and Campbell (1995) concludes that since 'whatever happened, nothing more could be done to harm or benefit Bland himself, it seems right to let the choice of outcome be decided by what would most benefit those closest to him.'

This, though, is a potentially dangerous principle. For it could mean that in some cases the wishes of relatives could be allowed to override those of the patient. For example, suppose the patient had made it clear to nursing and/or other health professional staff that, to whatever extent their mental capacity deteriorated, they would not want any action or inaction taken which might shorten their natural life. Then, when the state of their mind is such that they are no longer able to communicate their wishes, and the relatives request that all active treatment stop because they cannot bear to see their loved one in such a state, whose wishes should take precedence? The principle of respecting autonomy would seem to suggest that the patient's wishes should be paramount. Thus, while the Tony Bland case may have established some legal principles, it most certainly has not ended the ethical debate.

Advanced directives

It has been suggested in the preceding discussions that patients' values and wishes made known in advance should be taken into account if they are subsequently in a condition which prevents them from participating in the decision-making process. The notion of *advanced directives* is a more formalized way of enabling people to make known their wishes in advance. Advanced directives have no formal legal status in the United Kingdom; however, the Select Committee of the House of Lords (1994) concluded that legislation was unnecessary as doctors increasingly recognised their ethical obligations to comply with them.

The BMA (1993) advocates that advanced directives should be respected unless there is evidence that the patient has since altered their position, or that if the request was for treatment not clinically indicated, or the action would be illegal.

The first of these three exceptions clearly accords with the principle of autonomy, in that it respects the current wishes of the patient. The second and third acknowledge the fact that autonomy is never pure or absolute. The patient cannot require of the health professional that they act in a way which in their professional judgement is not appropriate. The health professional also has a right to moral autonomy. And, clearly no one can require another to act illegally. What this means is, for example that in the United Kingdom a person may not expect their expressed wishes for active euthanasia to be respected given that the act of deliberately ending life is illegal.

SUMMARY

In this chapter I have attempted to outline some of the main arguments surrounding a number of ethical issues associated with death and dying. In all these discussions I leave it to the reader to decide which is the stronger case. Is the case for active euthanasia stronger than that against? Should health professionals be able to make decisions about whom to resuscitate, or is there an argument for having hard and fast rules? Is there a case for overriding the wishes of a patient when they are no longer in a position to give consent? In all the issues raised in this chapter there are, of course, other arguments and viewpoints on which I have not touched, and these would require equally lengthy discussion. Hugh Trowell (1973) subtitled his book *The Unfinished Debate on Euthanasia*, and doubtless the debate on euthanasia and the other issues touched on here will continue for many years.

Issues for Discussion

In the Tony Bland case the court determined that artificial hydration and nutrition required medical intervention for its application and was widely regarded by the medical profession as medical treatment. Nursing, on the other hand, has long since regarded the maintenance of nutrition and the feeding of patients as lying within its domain. Henderson included it as one of her *components of nursing*, Orem includes it as one of the *universal self-care requisites*, and Roper *et al.* include it as one of the *activities of living*. All of the aforementioned along with many other nursing theorists consider helping patients meet their nutritional needs as being an essential element of nursing.

There are therefore two questions to be addressed. First, is the meeting of patients' nutritional requirements a medical or nursing responsibility? And, second, is there a significant difference between natural and artificial means of feeding? If the answer to the first is that it is a nursing responsibility, and to the second that there is no difference, where do nurses stand in the light of the judgement in the Tony Bland case?

REFERENCES

Aarons, E.J. & Beeching, N.J. (1991) Survey of 'Do not resuscitate' orders in a district general hospital. *British Medical Journal*, 303(14), December, 1504–1506.

Bandman, E.L. & Bandman, B. (1990) *Nursing Ethics through the Life Span*, 2nd edn. Englewood Cliffs, NJ: Prentice Hall.

British Medical Association (1981) *The Handbook of Medical Ethics*. London: BMA.

British Medical Association (1993) *Statement on Advanced Directives*. London: BMA.

Campbell, R. (1995) The critically ill patient, B An ethical perspective – declining and withdrawing treatment. In Tingle, J. & Cribb, A. (eds) (1995) *Nursing Law and Ethics*. Oxford: Blackwell Science, Ch. 9, pp. 218–229.

Fletcher, J. (1973) Ethics and euthanasia. *American Journal of Nursing*, 73(4), April.

House of Lords (1994) Paper 21, Vol 1: Report VII: Oral evidence; Vol III: Written evidence. London: HMSO.

Mitchell, K.R. *et al.* (1993) Medical futility, treatment withdrawal and the persistent vegetative state. *Journal of Medical Ethics*, 18, Supplement.

Montague, P. (1978) The morality of active and passive euthanasia. *Ethics in Science and Medicine*, 5, 39–45.

Nelson, J.B. (1973) *Human Medicine*. Minnesota: Augsberg Publishing House.

Rayner, The Most Rev. K. (1976) Euthanasia: a Christian perspective. *Australian and New Zealand Journal of Surgery*, 46(4), November.

Singleton, J. & McLaren, S. (1995) *Ethical Foundations of Health Care – Responsibilities in Decision-Making*. London: Mosby.

Stanley, J.M. (1992) Developing guidelines for decisions to forgo life-prolonging medical treatment. *Journal of Medical Ethics*, 18, Supplement.

Trowell, H. (1973) *Euthanasia – the Unfinished Debate on Euthanasia*. London: SCM.

UKCC (United Kingdom Central Council for Nursing, Midwifery and Health Visiting) (1989) *Exercising Accountability*. London: UKCC.

UKCC (United Kingdom Central Council for Nursing, Midwifery and Health Visiting) (1992) *Code of Professional Conduct for the Nurse, Midwife and Health Visitor*, 3rd edn. London: UKCC.

Weber, L.J. (1973) Ethics and euthanasia – another view. *American Journal of Nursing*, 73(7), July.

FURTHER READING

Church Information Office (1975) *On Dying Well*. London: Church Information Office.

Kubler-Ross, E. (1978) *To Live Until We Say Goodbye*. Englewood Cliffs, NJ: Prentice-Hall.

Saunders, C.M. (1975) Terminal care. In Bagshawe, K.D. (ed.) *Medical Oncology*. Oxford: Blackwell.

Singleton, J. & McLaren, S. (1995) *Ethical Foundations of Health Care – Responsibilities in Decision-Making*. London: Mosby.

See: Chapter 7, 'Acts and Omissions, the Doctrine of Double Effect, and Ordinary and Extraordinary Means'; Chapter 8, 'Critical Ethical Approach to the Problem of Euthanasia'; Chapter 9, 'Definitions of life and death'.

The Linacre Centre, *Linacre Centre Papers*: Prolongation of Life. Paper 2: 'Is there a Morally Significant Difference between Killing and Letting Die?' (1978); and Paper 3: 'Ordinary and Extraordinary Means of Prolonging Life' (1979).

8

The unborn child

In this chapter several issues related to the unborn child will be discussed; namely, abortion, artificial insemination, *in vitro* fertilization, embryo research and surrogate motherhood. Pertinent to all these issues is the question 'When does human life begin?', and that must be the starting point of our discussion.

THE BEGINNING OF HUMAN LIFE

To some extent the answer to the question will be affected by one's definition of human life and, as we saw in Chapters 4 and 7, there are various definitions. For the moment we can put the question of what constitutes human life to one side and turn to some facts. We know that the development of human life begins with the coming together of sperm and ovum and that it continues through life *in utero* to birth and beyond. 'The continuous and uninterrupted development of the *conceptus* into a new-born child suggests that human life is present from the moment of conception' (Varga, 1980). The moment of conception, then, is one answer to the question of when human life begins.

Others have argued that it begins at different stages of development – the implantation of the fertilized egg in the uterine wall, the commencement of brain activity, the beginning of spontaneous movements of the fetus, viability, even the moment of birth itself. All of these are signs of stages in development. They are all known to occur and can be identified in each individual. None in themselves can really lead one to the assumption that the nature of the fetus has changed, because they are nothing more than signs that the fetus has moved from one stage of biological development to the next. Why should, for example, a non-viable fetus be non-human and a viable one human? Identifying precisely the moment at which the fetus becomes viable is difficult, and what is considered viable today was not so 100, even 20, years ago. Hence the demand in 1990 to reform the Abortion Act of 1967. The debate which surrounded the reform of the Abortion Act was concerned chiefly with this question of viability. As a criterion for pinpointing the moment at which human life begins it is unreliable and illogical.

> *This capacity to survive independently is contingent upon technologies and interventions that, at this moment, make the point of viability somewhere in the area of 20 to 24 weeks in gestation. If, however, the point of viability were reduced technologically to a much earlier point, perhaps even to the point of conception, holders of the viability position would logically have to shift with the state of the art.*
>
> (Veatch, 1981)

Again, why should a viable fetus be non-human or a non-person but a new-born child a person? While science provides us with valuable information about the development of a human being from conception to birth and beyond, it cannot pinpoint the moment at which personhood begins. The reason being that, with one possible exception, biological viability, those attributes which are said to be essential elements of personhood are not measurable by scientific means. If, as was suggested in Chapter 4, a 'person' is someone who exhibits a level of rationality, sentience and the capacity to feel and experience sensation and express desires and wishes, then that those elements are present in the unborn child is to some extent supposition.

However, there is growing evidence to suggest that a fetus experiences pain at a very early stage in development. Until recently it had been thought that awareness and sentience were solely functions of the cerebral cortex. However, 'growing evidence shows that the thalamus (the lower part of the brain which develops early in gestation) probably plays a more crucial role in consciousness than was previously recognised.' (Peacock, 1997). And, Professor Christopher Hull (1997) states, 'So far as I am concerned, I would be prepared to accept that foetuses do not experience pain when somebody proves to me that they don't feel pain. But until that time, I would have to assume that they do.'

It would seem then that a considerable number of the attributes which constitute personhood exist in the fetus at an early stage. We know that at a very early stage the fetus possesses all the anatomical components which make up a human being, and evidence now suggests that at an early stage it also possesses sentience and the capacity to feel and experience sensations.

The one attribute which we cannot measure in the unborn is the ability for rational thinking or reasoning. Actual possession of the ability to reason can be tested, but only once the child has developed communication skills to such a level as to be able to demonstrate that ability. Indeed, some would argue that the ability to reason occurs at quite a late stage in development, and one is left with the obviously nonsensical idea that full personhood occurs at some stage after birth. If, on the other hand, what distinguishes human life from non-human life is the possession of a soul or spirit, then again we cannot know whether or not the soul is in the unborn child. There is no scientific measurement or test for its existence. To some extent we cannot be certain until a later stage in a child's development that it possesses all the attributes of personhood, and only then can we say retrospectively that the potential was there all along. The question 'when does life begin?' is not a scientific one but a philosophical one.

What answers do philosophers have to offer? As one would expect, philosophers agree about this no more than scientists do. At one time Catholic theologians claimed that *ensoulment* occurred at the moment the fertilized egg became implanted in the uterine wall. Few, if any, modern Catholic theologians would be so definite.[1] The trend of thought would seem to be that, since ensoulment occurs at some unidentifiable stage, it is better to err on the side of safety and assume that is at the earliest possible moment.

Essentially, the argument is whether it is the potential to develop or actual possession of those attributes which constitute personhood that determines that a being is a person. If we follow the development of the fetus in reverse, beginning with the point of birth, then it is difficult to identify in what way the essential nature of the fetus has changed at each stage. The fetus immediately pre-birth is exactly the same as that which emerges at the time of birth. And so, we can backtrack through all the stages of fetal development. Nothing enters the fetus at any point to bring about the next stage of development.

Take, for example, the commencement of electrical activity in the brain. This occurs naturally as part of the growth cycle. One cannot claim that, because cessation of brain activity is synonymous with death, before brain activity begins there is no life, when clearly there is. 'The developing embryo has the natural capacity to bring on the functioning of the brain' (Varga, 1980). For the brain to start functioning there must already be life present. It is not the brain but something else which provides the impetus.

Throughout development it is something already present which sparks off the change or the next stage. Thus we begin to see that there is something in the embryo itself which starts the development of all human activities. It seems logical therefore to take as the starting point of *human life* the time of conception, for that is the point at which two hitherto separate entities (namely, the sperm and the ovum) come together to make a new entity which is potentially a new-born child. 'There comes a point where the personhood of the fetus is either an article of faith or it is not' (Campbell, 1975). The argument that human life begins with fertilization may not be totally convincing, and, like most philosophical arguments, it cannot be proved in the way that, for example, a law of physics can.

Nevertheless, it has enough weight to establish at least the probability of the presence of a human individual at conception. This probability in turn substantiates the duty not to expose the developing fetus to danger or to deliberately kill it, because we are obliged to choose the safer course and to avoid harming a being that is possibly or probably human.

(Varga, 1980)

The argument may appear very tortuous, but we do need to try to establish the point at which human life begins before we can begin to discuss ethical issues related to the unborn child. Clearly, if one were able with certainty to pinpoint a stage in development at which human life began – say, viability – then one could argue that there would be no need to afford to the unviable fetus the respect and rights we afford to a human being. The question of the morality of abortion pre-viability would possibly not arise.

ABORTION

In most ethical debates there are those who see everything in clear terms of black and white, and those who see a varying number of shades of grey. In this the issue of abortion is typical. The positions taken range from those who say the act of abortion is an act of killing and therefore wrong, through those who take the view that it may be permitted in certain circumstances, to those who take the view that there is nothing at all immoral in the act. We shall look first at the two extreme positions, and then discuss some of the grey areas in between.

The arguments against abortion

Put simply, the argument against abortion is based on two moral assumptions; firstly, that it is wrong to kill a human being; secondly, that the unborn child is a human being and therefore has the same *right to life* as any other human being. There is, as we have already seen, debate as to when human life begins. Consequently, there are those who say that abortion is wrong at any stage, since human life begins at the moment of conception, while others would argue that it becomes morally wrong only at the point at which they contend that human life begins. Therefore, in discussing the arguments against abortion we are not concerned with the stage of development up to which abortion may be condoned, but with the arguments against killing what, regardless of the stage of development, is contended to be a human life.

As already stated, the basic argument is that to take a human life is wrong, therefore to take the life of a fetus is wrong. And, as we shall see later, this contention is adhered to even when to allow the fetus to continue to birth may have undesirable consequences either for the mother or the child. The chief moral dilemma which anti-abortionists have to face is when a choice has to be made between saving the life of the fetus and saving the life of the mother. The reason that it is a dilemma is because one is then faced with a choice between two courses of action, both of which will result in an undesirable outcome – the ending of a human life.

It is rare today that such a choice has to be made. With the advances in obstetrics, probably the only cases in which such a decision arises are those of ectopic pregnancies, and even in these cases the decision is fairly clear cut. Whichever course of action is chosen, the fetus will almost certainly die, and the choice is actually between destroying one life, that of the fetus, and risking the lives of both fetus and mother.

If a situation arises in which a choice does have to be made between the life of the mother and the life of the unborn child, then one would have to decide which life is of the greater value. Campbell (1975) argues that 'It is difficult to see how the life of the fetus and the life of the mother can be regarded on an equal footing, far less that the fetus be given priority'. One cannot do otherwise than agree with Campbell, for how can the mother's life, a life which already exists in its fullness, be equated with the life of a fetus, which may or may not come to fruition?

On the other hand, LIFE (1994) argue that even in those rare situations where the life of the mother is threatened by the pregnancy, as this usually occurs late in pregnancy, there is no reason to perform an abortion – to kill the child. They agree that the pregnancy should be ended, to prevent the death of both mother and child, but argue that the child be delivered by surgery and given a chance to survive.

So far the discussion has been based on the assumption that the fetus is a human life. However, some anti-abortionists would argue that even if it is not a human life it is potentially a human life and should be treated in the same way.

The argument in favour of abortion

As we shall see later, there are several arguments put forward to justify abortion in particular circumstances. First, however, we consider the case put forward by those who see no objection to abortion under any circumstances – the case for abortion on demand. The argument is that a woman has rights over her own body and therefore should have a right to an abortion if, for whatever reason, she does not want to bear a child. The main argument is based on the notion of the *right to privacy*. 'Respect for privacy is the basis for the concern that the pregnant woman maintain control over her own body' (Fenner, 1980). If we accept the notion that, in other contexts, patients have the right to determine what shall be done to their bodies, then why should that notion not also apply to a pregnant woman? The argument would seem to be particularly strong with respect to the woman whose pregnancy is not of her choosing.

Furthermore, in some circumstances, particularly when the pregnancy is the result of rape or incest, the quality of life of the mother may be severely harmed, and the quality of life of the 'unwanted' child may be minimal. Pro-abortionists would argue that *quality of life* is equally as important as *right to life*, and that by over-valuing life *per se* the quality of all life comes into question. However, the question is, can one reasonably equate the *value* of one life with the *quality* of another?

Abortion in specific situations – a question of values

As has already been indicated, much of the discussion about abortion is to do with comparing the *value* of the developing human life with some other value. In each case one has to decide which is the greater: the value of the fetus or the conflicting value.

The 1967 Abortion Act[2] gives the following as grounds for abortion:

1. That the continuance of the pregnancy would involve risk to the life of the pregnant woman or of injury to the physical or mental health of the pregnant woman, or of any existing children of her family, greater than if the pregnancy were terminated.
2. That there is a substantial risk that if the child were born it would suffer from such physical or mental abnormalities as to be severely handicapped.

The values, then, with which the life of the fetus is being compared are:

◆ the life of the mother;
◆ the quality of life of the mother;
◆ the quality of life of siblings;
◆ the potential quality of its own life.

The main issue is that, apart from in the first instance, we are dealing with unequal values. For can we really equate the value of life with quality of life? This, as we shall see, is central to the argument surrounding the justification of abortion in specific instances. And it is to those specific instances that we now turn.

Therapeutic abortion

We have already, albeit briefly, dealt with those rare occasions in which the decision which has to be made is between the life of the mother and the life of the fetus. More commonly, the decision concerns the effects on the mother's health or quality of life in proceeding with the pregnancy. Advocates of therapeutic abortion would argue that the physical health of the pregnant woman is more valuable than the life of the fetus. Thus they would justify the act on the grounds that the greater value has been chosen. There are problems with this kind of justification. Firstly, as Varga (1980) argues, human life is more valuable than physical health and, secondly, there remains the question as to whether the abortion is necessary to restore health. Most complications of pregnancy can be dealt with by modern medicine. Illness arising during, but not caused by, pregnancy will not be cured by abortion and, whenever possible, if pregnancy intensifies the illness, remedies should be applied until the fetus reaches viability. There is no suggestion that either the health of the mother might not suffer as a result of the pregnancy or that the physical health is not of higher value. The argument is that the life of the fetus is of greater value than the physical health of the mother and that remedies other than abortion should be sought to improve the mother's health. The same basic argument, according to Varga, applies when the pregnancy affects the mental health of the mother.

What, then, of the contention in the Abortion Act 1967 that abortion is justified on the grounds that the continuance of the pregnancy would be harmful to any existing children? The argument here is based on the utilitarian principle of the greatest happiness for the greatest number. It can be argued that, if as a result of the pregnancy and subsequent birth, the health and well-being of existing children will suffer, then abortion is justified. Although the ending of the pregnancy will be of no benefit to the fetus other children, it will result in, at least, the prevention of harm to them. The arrival in a large family of an additional, perhaps unwanted, child will clearly have an effect on all concerned. The existing children may well suffer as a result of meagre resources having to be spread further and from a loss of attention from their mother. The new arrival might also have a less than ideal existence. The argument against abortion on such grounds is two-fold. Firstly, one can only conjecture the effect of the arrival of an additional child, and, secondly, it is to equate the value of human happiness and well-being with the value of human life.

Before moving on to the second main reason given in the Abortion Act for justifying abortion – the risk that the unborn child will be severely handicapped – we will consider one other frequently posed justification, which relates more to the health and well-being of the mother.

Rape and incest

It is commonly argued that abortion is justified when the pregnancy occurs as a result of rape or incest. This is a very sensitive and emotive area, and in attempting to discuss objectively the morality of abortion in such situations, we must be careful not to appear insensitive to the very real sufferings of women and girls who are victims of rape or incest. While there is a very clear moral and legal distinction to be made between rape and incest, here it is assumed that the incestuous act was entered into involuntarily on the part of the woman or girl, and that therefore any resulting pregnancy can be viewed in the same way as a pregnancy arising from the act of rape.

It is argued that abortion under these circumstances is justified for three reasons: firstly, that abortion will safeguard the mental health of the woman, which is undoubtedly at risk and of great value; secondly, that pregnancy resulting from rape or incest is a grave injustice and that the victim is therefore under no obligation to carry the fetus to viability; and finally, it is sometimes argued that the fetus is an aggressor against the woman's personal life and integrity, and that it is morally defensible to repel an aggressor, even by killing him or her in order to protect human values.

The third argument carries less weight than the other two. The fetus is not the aggressor. It is the perpetrator of the rape who is the aggressor, and the fetus is as much the innocent victim of the act as is the woman. The destruction of the fetus cannot be justified on this ground.

The strict, objective moral argument against abortion in such cases on the grounds of the effects it will have on the mental well-being of the mother is that the value of human life 'has to be placed higher on the scale of values than the values a woman could obtain by abortion' (Varga, 1980). However, society clearly has a moral duty towards rape victims and should offer to them far more in terms of psychological help and support than it frequently does. On humane grounds, unless there is adequate support, then abortion appears to be a reasonable solution. Sadly, the psychological effects of an abortion may well compound rather than alleviate those of rape.

Eugenic abortion

Eugenic abortion is abortion of a fetus which if allowed to survive would result in a child with severe physical or mental handicap. The handicapping condition may, for example, be caused by viral infections such as exposure to rubella during the first trimester, the use of certain drugs during pregnancy (thalidomide was a tragic instance), or due to genetic defects (Down's syndrome being one of the commonest). It is argued that it is better for a child not to be born than to lead a life burdened with a crippling disorder.

Modern medical advances, such as amniocentesis, have made it possible to identify an abnormal fetus at an early stage and therefore made possible abortion at a stage permitted in law. As our ability to identify more and more abnormalities at an increasingly early stage improves, so the question of abortion as a solution is more frequently quently raised. 'Some eugenicists would even make it obligatory to destroy seriously defective life before birth. As it stands now eugenic abortion is legal in most countries but not obligatory' (Varga, 1980). As has been argued elsewhere in this book, the ability to do something or the fact that an act is legal does not mean that it is morally right. What then is the morality of eugenic abortion?

It is argued that eugenic abortion is primarily for the benefit of the child and only secondarily for the benefit of the parents. This argument is a false one. The abortion is not for the benefit of the patient, who is the child. Abortion will not cure his disease but destroy him. It could be argued that ending the child's life before it has really begun is preventing a life of suffering and misery and that it does benefit him. In so arguing, one is weighing the value of life itself against the value accorded to the quality of that life. Even if one claims that is a justifiable balancing of values, one still has the problem of measuring the unknown – the quality of a life which is as yet still developing. Just as we saw in Chapter 4 that it is very difficult to assess the quality of life of someone who cannot communicate their feelings, so it is impossible to assess the quality of life of an unborn child.

The other argument is that, in preventing the birth of a severely handicapped child, one is avoiding the hardships and suffering that caring for the child would place on the family, and the expense to society in meeting the child's and family's needs. Here, as in the case of therapeutic abortions, one is balancing two unequal values – the life of a human being against the suffering of others.

Against all of this we have the evidence that many children born with severe handicaps live enjoyable and worthwhile lives. Furthermore:

> *Our social nature imposes a duty upon us and the whole society to look after the less fortunate members of the human family. That many persons understand this obligation of our common humanity is indicated by the fact that the number of couples adopting victims of genetic defects has been growing rapidly.*

> (Varga, 1980)

ARTIFICIAL INSEMINATION

Until the last decade or so, most of us probably thought that artificial insemination was something that veterinary surgeons did to cows. This practice aroused little ethical debate. However, what has now become a reality is artificial insemination of women, and this practice has aroused much ethical debate. There are two categories of artificial insemination – artificial insemination by husband and artificial insemination by donor. These give rise to three moral stands. Firstly, that neither is morally acceptable; secondly, that artificial insemination by husband is acceptable, while that by donor is not; and thirdly, that both are acceptable.

Essentially, then, there are two questions which have to be addressed. Firstly, is artificial insemination morally acceptable? Secondly, if it is, are there any moral distinctions to be made between artificial insemination by husband and artificial insemination by donor? Obviously the second question arises only if the answer to the first is 'Yes'.

We begin, therefore, by addressing the question 'Is artificial insemination morally acceptable?'. The question has less to do with the question posed at the beginning of this chapter, 'When does human life begin?', and more to do with differing definitions of marriage and parenthood. The Catholic position is that artificial insemination by husband or donor for reasons of sterility or fallopian tube closure is morally wrong.

> ...*artificial insemination is an act of production rather than communion between two people. [It] reduces human beings to objects and degrades their being, value, and dignity. Married couples have no right to children, only the right to perform the procreative act.*

> (Berger, 1987)

While one can accept the logic of the argument, there does seem to be some degree of contradiction here with the traditional Catholic teaching on marriage and procreation (see Ch. 3). It is claimed that the purpose of marriage is the procreation of children, and one of the arguments against contraception is that it prevents procreation. Yet, here the argument is that a procedure which enables procreation, and thus enables the couple to fulfil their duty, is wrong. Of course, this is to over-simplify the issue. For what lies at the heart of the objections to contraception and artificial insemination is that both are *artificial* acts, and both are intended to thwart the course of nature.

Essentially, the arguments against and for artificial insemination revolve around whether the acts of sexual intercourse, procreation and child-rearing can or cannot be separated. If procreation is seen as a continuous process beginning with the sexual act and ending with a mature, independent being, then there can be no separation of the various elements of that process. On the other hand, if the elements are seen as being not necessarily connected, and capable of being judged in isolation, then there is a case for arguing that artificial insemination is acceptable. For if the act of sexual intercourse is seen as being primarily an expression of love between two people, it can be seen as an end in itself. Procreation then also becomes a process begun for its own sake. Therefore, it can be argued that if a couple who, for one reason or another, are incapable of producing a child by natural means and are desirous to create and nurture a child, they have the right to do so.

> *The human acts of sexual intimacy and procreation are different and separate. The main argument is that parenthood is not primarily a matter of biology but instead a broadly human function of commitment to the care and rearing of a child.*

(Bandman and Bandman, 1990)

This answers the question of whether artificial insemination by husband might be acceptable, but what of artificial insemination by donor?

If we accept the notion that a couple has the right to rear a child, but if due to some physiological impairment they are unable to create for themselves a fertilized ovum, do they have the right to rear a child which is not the result of their own conceiving? That a couple who are incapable of producing a child of their own are nevertheless entitled to nurture a child is a long-accepted idea, for that is precisely what occurs when a couple adopt a child. Indeed, it is seen as a morally commendable thing to do in many circumstances, since it provides a secure family environment for an otherwise parentless child. Herein, perhaps, lies the essential point. When a childless couple adopt an orphaned child, they are doing something to benefit the child. This is quite different from artificial insemination by donor. For in artificial insemination by donor the motivation is not to provide a family for a child, but to provide a child to satisfy the desires of the parents. It is, in effect, to treat the unborn child as a product.

There are a number of objections raised to the use of artificial insemination by donor (AID), of which the following are the most frequently expressed. AID may not be acceptable to both partners and so lead to tensions and division between them. However, one would hope that before entering into the programme, both partners would have been counselled and given fully informed consent. Of more concern, perhaps, are the consequent effects on the child. The parents may keep the child's origin secret and so deny them the right to fundamental information about their existence. Or, the child must live with the knowledge that their biological father may never be known, and that their nurturing parents deliberately involved a third part to create pregnancy.

IN VITRO FERTILIZATION

In vitro fertilization (IVF) is the process by which an ovum is removed from a woman's body, mixed with the sperm of her partner, and placed in a growth medium. Fertilization then occurs, and after a period of 10–14 days the blastocyst (the eight-cell stage) is implanted in the woman's uterus and, it is hoped, the pregnancy proceeds as normal. The procedure was first successfully performed in the United Kingdom in 1978.

The ethical debate surrounding IVF is wide-ranging, and not, as we shall see, dissimilar to that concerning artificial insemination. Some argue that 'it is unnatural and undermines the marriage covenant of sexual love for procreation' (Bandman and Bandman, 1990). The argument is, as was alluded to in the previous section, that child-rearing is a continuous process which begins with sexual intercourse and ends when the child grows to maturity and moves away from the parents to live a fully independent adult life. To separate the sexual act of procreation from the rest of this ongoing process is to treat the sexual act of procreation 'as a mere biological function, and defines parenthood as nurturing life, not generating life' (McCormick, 1978). This argument might hold if it were agreed that the sole purpose of sexual intercourse was procreation. However, if the act is seen as an end in itself, as an expression of love, and not always undertaken with the intention of creating life, then there is no logical reason for claiming that the sexual act of procreation and the nurturing of a child, both within and beyond the womb, cannot be separated.

A further concern is that of risk of damage to the embryo which could result in an abnormal baby. The risk is not thought to be great, but there is still uncertainty about how great or slight it might be. The question of whether or not to take the risk has to be decided by the couple, but as Fromer (1981) points out, because of lack of knowledge they are not able to make an *informed* decision; their decision will be a more or less blind one. The key question is whether the risk of damage is greater than that which occurs during the course of nature. In other words, is there a greater risk of damage occurring between IVF and implantation than there is between the time of natural fertilization and implantation? Some moral philosophers and scientists argue that even if the risk is only slightly increased, then it is morally unacceptable.

IVF also involves the question of rights. 'A barren couple has the right to take action and to use available technology to counteract that barrenness' (Fromer, 1981). If IVF represents a couple's only possible hope of counteracting their barrenness, then IVF comes to be seen as a *therapeutic* rather than *experimental* procedure. Equally, the doctor has the right to give what he or she considers to be the most appropriate therapy to a barren couple as to any 'patient'. One could even claim that the doctor has a duty so to do. Therefore, it is argued, the decision involves the couple and the doctor, and neither the State nor any other outside body has the right to interfere.

Then there is the question of what rights, if any, the blastocyst has. This takes us back to the earlier debate about when human life begins. If one takes the view that human life begins with implantation, then clearly the blastocyst cannot be considered an entity and therefore has no rights. If, on the other hand, one takes the view that human life begins with fertilization, then the minute collection of cells which begins to form *in vitro* from the moment of fertilization must be treated with the respect due to a human being.

The concern of most moralists is not so much with the procedure of IVF itself as with some of the developments that could arise from it. At the moment it is not possible to support the growth of an embryo outside the uterus much beyond the blastocyst stage, still less bring it to full term. The fear of some moralists is that in time it will be possible that there will be such a thing as an artificial womb. Already scientists have laid claim to supporting the development of an embryo to 59 days (Varga, 1980). The embryo has by this time reached a stage of development not normally achieved until after implantation. Is it human or not?

The possibility of growing babies in the laboratory is still very much in the future, but IVF does make other developments possible, and it is to some of those developments that we now turn.

Surrogate motherhood

In IVF the woman's ovum is removed, fertilized, and then implanted in her own uterus. The natural development of this procedure has been the transfer of an embryo. It is now possible for doctors to implant the ovum fertilized *in vitro* in the uterus of another woman or to transplant an embryo from the uterus of one woman to that of another. There are two distinct types of surrogacy, namely *partial*, also known as *traditional* or *straight* surrogacy, and *full*, also known as *host* or *IVF* surrogacy. In *partial* surrogacy, the surrogate mother provides the egg. The sperm from the intended father is placed into the surrogate mother's vagina, either by the mother herself or a health professional, and fertilization then takes place in the usual way. In *full* surrogacy usually the sperm and ova of the intended parents are fertilized in vitro and the fertilized ova (usually one or two) are placed in the uterus of the surrogate mother. There are two further variations of this procedure. If the intended father is infertile then the intended mother's ova may be fertilized *in vitro* by sperm from a donor, or if the intended mother is infertile then the father's sperm may be used to fertilize the ova from a donor.

Clearly, surrogacy offers childless couples a tremendous hope. However, the various types of surrogacy raise differing issues. In the case of partial surrogacy only the father has a genetic link with the child. The intended mother has no genetic link but the surrogate mother does and this can lead to later conflict. Not least because, in the United Kingdom, surrogacy arrangements are not enforceable in law and the legal mother is always the carrying mother (i.e. the surrogate mother). That the surrogate mother is genetically linked to the child may cause her to be more inclined to want to keep the child once she has given birth. The problems noted earlier as arising from AID would also apply as they would in cases of full surrogacy where only one of the intended parents has a genetic link with the child. In the case of full surrogacy where the sperm and ova from the intended parents are used, other than the legal status of the child, there are likely to be fewer objections. The child, although carried by, and delivered of another woman would genetically be theirs. 'One could argue that it respects human life and that it is only good medicine to help childless couples to have their own genetic children.' (Varga, 1980), a view supported by the BMA (1996).

However, some ethicists of the natural law school would argue that all forms of surrogacy are contrary to natural law, that it is an interference with natural biological processes. Such an argument is rather weak inasmuch as a great deal of medical intervention is an interference with natural processes. To argue that interference in some instances is wrong and in others is right is clearly illogical.

Two issues which arise from the possibility of surrogate motherhood and which are of great concern to moralists are the use of the procedure for convenience rather than necessity, and payment of the surrogate mother.

Suppose an unmarried woman, who is committed to her career, wishes to raise a child. She does not, however, wish to interrupt her career by becoming pregnant. She could enlist the services of another woman to carry her child. The argument against such an idea revolves around the concept of motherhood. There is a distinction between the woman who desperately wants a child but for some medical reason is unable either to conceive or carry a child to full term, and one who is quite able to do so but for reasons of convenience chooses not to. Some would question the woman's motives in having a child, for it might seem that the child is being brought into existence for purely selfish reasons and not for his or her own sake as a person, but this might equally well be said of children born naturally to some parents. We should not assume that because a woman elects not to bear her own child that she will not care for and value that child when it is born.

The more fundamental argument against surrogacy is that which was raised in the earlier discussion about artificial insemination: that it separates the act of procreation from child-rearing. This would, of course, apply equally to the case of the infertile couple as to that of the woman who chooses not to bear her own child. Again, as in the earlier debate, the argument is easily refuted.

The idea of payment being made to surrogate mothers is abhorrent to many. It has long been established, since the abolition of slavery, that human beings are not a saleable commodity. It could, on the other hand, be argued that a couple were not *buying* the child from the surrogate mother, but simply paying her for nurturing it from the moment of implantation to the time of birth, and that there is no difference between that and paying a nanny or child-minder to care for the child after birth. The BMA (1996) sees no objections to payment being made to surrogate mothers for expenses, citing the figure of £7,000 to £10,000.

Of greater concern to moralists is the notion of payment being made to a third party, such as an agent for surrogacy. To commercialize what is seen as being a humane service, and to make a profit out of the need and sufferings of childless couples, is abhorrent to many. It is argued that, just as for adoption, the surrogacy arrangements should be made by the State or a voluntary organization who have at interest the needs of the parents and the child. The treatment of infertility can be viewed in the same way as the treatment of other health problems, and is something to which people have a right. The ability to exercise that right should not be determined by the ability to pay.

Donation of ovum

A further development of the principle of embryo transfer is donation of ovum. Suppose a woman is unable to ovulate or to produce healthy ova. She could be helped in one of three ways. The ovum of another woman could be fertilized by her husband either by artificial insemination or *in vitro*, and the fertilized ovum implanted in the *sterile* woman. Alternatively, the ovum of another woman could be transferred to the sterile woman and then fertilized *in vivo* by her husband. The child, when born, would be the genetic child of only one partner, the husband, and a third party. The moral argument against such a procedure is that a third person is introduced into the marriage which is contrary to the notion that a marriage is by nature the exclusive relationship of one man and one woman. The same argument is used against artificial insemination by donor, not the husband.

Underlying the concerns about IVF and embryo transfer is the question of the safety of the procedure both to the child and the mother. Dr Steptoe is reported as saying that the birth of Louise Brown[3] came only after 'roughly a hundred unsuccessful efforts' (Varga, 1980). At present, embryo transfer involves the destruction of several embryos. If human life begins at the time of fertilization, then such a practice is unethical because it involves the destruction of human life. And this, as we shall see, is central to the debate about embryo research.

EMBRYO RESEARCH

'It has been suggested that tampering with the embryo is itself unethical. This problem arises from the lack of agreement as to when human life begins' (Royal College of Nursing, 1983). The questions of what status we afford to and how we treat an embryo, in or outside of the uterus, depends very much on at what stage in development we consider that human life begins. If we accept the notion that human life begins at conception, then an embryo is a human life. If, on the other hand, we take the line that human life begins with implantation, then we have a very different scenario. In terms of embryo research, and in particular when the embryo has been created *in vitro*, then both these points of view pose questions about the morality of research on embryos.

If we accept the idea that human life begins at the time of conception – namely, the point at which the ovum is fertilized by a sperm – then all embryos are human lives. And, if that is the case, should we treat it with the same respect as we would any other human life? If the answer is 'Yes', then we must apply the same rules to experimentation on embryos as we apply to humans at any other stage of development. 'One has to conclude that the bringing into existence and destruction of human embryos for the sake of research is unethical' (Varga, 1980).

However, can we actually equate an embryo which has been created artificially – that is, by the bringing together of sperm and ovum in a laboratory setting – with one created naturally by the bringing together of sperm and ovum within a woman's body through the act of sexual intercourse? This is a very crucial question. For, at whatever stage we consider that human life begins, an essential element must surely be that it is the product of human sexual intercourse.

If we accept the notion that human life begins at the point of implantation, then an embryo created *in vitro* cannot until it is implanted in a uterus be considered a human life. In this case, it can be treated as any other laboratory substance, and not subject to any rules which might be applied to experimentation on humans. This might seem to present no problem. But what if it becomes possible to keep alive in a laboratory situation an embryo which is older than the stage at which in normal situations implantation would occur? Is it then a human being or not? The same question arises if the beginning of human life is believed to occur at some later stage of development, such as *quickening* or the onset of electrical activity in the brain.

One way of answering the question might be to say that any embryo is a *potential* human life, and therefore should be treated as if it were a human life. The major problem associated with the *potential human life* argument is at what point do you stop? For, essentially, every sperm and every ovum is a potential human life. This is, of course one of the arguments put forward against those forms of contraception which seek to destroy either the sperm or the ovum. However, since not every ovum, and by no means every sperm, can ever develop into an embryo, let alone a child, this is clearly an illogical line of argument.

Assuming that an embryo is either a human life or potential human life, what are the arguments for and against embryo research? One argument put forward by proponents of research on embryos is that it is justifiable because it is undertaken for one of two main reasons: firstly, to perfect existing or develop new procedures for helping apparently infertile couples; and secondly, to discover ways of preventing congenital or hereditary disorders.

They would argue that the benefits to be obtained from embryo research are sufficient to justify bringing embryos into existence for the purpose of research even if it results in the destruction of the embryo. However, if human life is present (or potentially present) in the embryo, it is difficult to see how any benefits, however great, can justify the creation of embryos solely for the purposes of experimentation and with almost certainty of destruction.

Suppose that an embryo was brought into existence, not primarily for the purpose of research but with the intention that it should be implanted and allowed to develop naturally to birth. Suppose, too, that it was possible to carry out research without endangering its life. If the embryo is a human life then research on it, given the conditions just described, can be justified only if it complies with the criteria pertaining to experimentation on human beings; namely, that the experimentation will not harm the subject and is designed to benefit him or her.[4] Benefit to others should be only a secondary outcome and not the prime purpose for the research. In the case of most research carried out on embryos the main purpose is to benefit others, and there is a high risk of harm being done to the subject.

SUMMARY

In all ethical issues relating to the unborn child the underlying question is 'When does human life begin?'. As we have seen, it is difficult, if not impossible, to state categorically at what stage in its development the unborn child becomes a human person. It seems therefore prudent to err on the side of safety and assume that human life begins at the moment of fertilization. That being so, when discussing issues involving the unborn child, we must assume that we are dealing with a human life. A second essential element is whether the act of child-rearing is a continuous one, beginning with sexual intercourse and ending with a fully independent mature being, or whether the sexual act, procreation and child-nurturing can be separated.

In this chapter some of the main arguments surrounding the more common issues have been discussed. There are other issues – for example, eugenics and genetic engineering – of which space does not allow discussion here. However, it is hoped that the reader has been provided with a framework on which to base discussion on these and other issues.

The concern in this chapter has been with the ethics of the acts themselves. In Chapter 16 we shall discuss the rights of the nurse when asked to participate in procedures, such as abortion, which he or she might hold to be morally wrong, and duties towards patients undergoing such procedures.

Issues for Discussion

Advances in IVF have given rise to a number of cases, particularly involving surrogacy, which presumably were not, and probably could not have been foreseen by early pioneers of this procedure. They raise questions, not so much about the ethics of the procedure itself as about its use and the need for controls.

What are the issues raised by the following cases? Do they suggest that tighter or more lenient controls are needed or that the whole idea of IVF and surrogacy should be reconsidered?

CASE 1

It was reported in the Daily Mail, March 1997, that an Italian surrogate mother was carrying babies for two separate sets of parents at the same time. Both fell into the category of full surrogacy with the sperm and ova of each pair of intended parents being used. The Italian gynecologist who performed the implantation said: 'I synchronized the ovulation of all three women and at the precisely correct moment implanted the embryos. Each is in a separate sac and will not interfere with each other.'

CASE 2

In 1996 Edith Jones gave birth to a child by caesarian section. She had been implanted with two embryos created from fertilized eggs from her daughter and son-in-law. At the time a spokesman for the Catholic Media Office said: 'This situation technically makes both the natural mother and the child of the same generation. It will surely cause considerable confusion to both children.'

Would your response to this case be different if the ova had been Edith's and not her daughter's?

CASE 3

In the United Kingdom the frozen sperm of a woman's deceased husband can be used for AIF (artificial insemination by father) or to fertilize her ova in vitro provided he has given written consent. Diane Blood's husband died unexpectedly from meningitis, before he could give written consent to his sperm being used. The Human Fertilisation and Embryology Authority ruled, and they were supported by the High Court, not to let her have fertility treatment at home or abroad. Apart from the humane issues involved, this case also raises questions about informed consent and whether legal and ethical principles are contingent or absolutes that need to be defended at whatever cost to actual living people.

NOTES

1. See the Declaration on Procured Abortion: Sacra Conregatio pro Doctrina Fidei (1974), 'Declaratio di aborto procurato', *Acta Apostolicae Sedis*, pp. 730–747.
2. As noted earlier, the changes made in 1990 to the Abortion Act were concerned largely with the stage at which an abortion might be carried out. Little change was made to other aspects of the 1967 Act, including conditions which justify an abortion.
3. The birth of Louise Brown was the culmination of many years' experimentation by Dr Robert Edwards and Dr Patrick Steptoe. Previously, in 1959, Dr Daniele Petrucci, an Italian geneticist and biologist, claimed to have successfully fertilized a human ovum *in vitro* and kept the developing embryo alive for 29 days, after which he destroyed it because it had become deformed. In 1974, Dr Douglas Bevis of Leeds University, England, announced that he had successfully implanted human ova, fertilized in test tubes, in the wombs of three women who had given birth to healthy babies. Despite Dr Bevis's bona fide reputation as a researcher, scientists are unwilling to accept his claim because of the immense veil of secrecy he drew over the identity of the women and babies.
4. See Chapter 9, in which experimentation on human beings is discussed more fully.

REFERENCES

Bandman, E.L. & Bandman, B. (1990) *Nursing Ethics through the Life Span.* Englewood Cliffs, NJ: Prentice-Hall.

Berger, J. (1987) Vatican official assails method of fertilization. *New York Times,* 8 October, B6; cited in Bandman, E.L. & Bandman, B. *Nursing Ethics through the Life Span.* Englewood Cliffs, NJ: Prentice-Hall.

British Medical Association (1996) *Changing Conceptions of Motherhood: the practice of surrogacy in Britain.* London: BMA.

Campbell, A.V. (1975) *Moral Dilemmas in Medicine.* Edinburgh: Churchill Livingstone.

Fenner, K.M. (1980) *Ethics and Law in Nursing: Professional Perspectives.* New York: Van Nostrand.

Fromer, M.J. (1981) *Ethical Issues in Health Care.* St Louis: C.V. Mosby.

Hull, C. (1997) cited by Peacock, E. (1977) In Donnellan, C. (ed.) *The Abortion Debate.* Issues for the Nineties, Vol. 34. Cambridge: Independence.

LIFE (1994) Hard questions answered. In Donnellan, C. (ed). *The Abortion Debate.* Issues for the Nineties, Vol. 34. Cambridge: Independence.

McCormick, R.A. (1978) Reproductive technologies: ethical issues. In Reich, W.T. (ed.) *Encyclopedia of Bioethics,* Vol. 4. New York: Free Press.

Peacock, E. (1997) The abortion debate. In Donnellan, C. (ed.) *The Abortion Debate.* Issues for the Nineties, Vol. 34. Cambridge: Independence.

Royal College of Nursing (1983) the unborn generations – humanity or convenience? *Nursing Mirror,* 1 June, 23–29.

Varga, A.C. (1980) *The Main Issues in Bioethics.* New York: Paulist Press.

Veatch, R.M. (1981) *A Theory of Medical Ethics.* New York: Basic Books.

FURTHER READING

Bandman, E.L. & Bandman, B. (1990) *Nursing Ethics through the Life Span.* Englewood Cliffs, NJ: Prentice-Hall.

See in particular Chapters 7, 'Nursing Ethics in the Procreative Family', and 8, 'Nursing Ethics and the Problem of Abortion'.

Fromer, M. (1981) *Ethical Issues in Health Care.* St Louis: C.V. Mosby.

See Chapter 3, 'Genetic Manipulatin': Chapter 4, 'Over-population'; Chapter 5, 'Artificial Insemination'; Chapter 7, 'Abortion'.

Donnellan, C. (ed.) (1997) *Surrogacy and IVF.* Issues for the Nineties, Vol. 11. Cambridge: Independence.

Donnellan, C. (ed.) (1997) *The Abortion Debate.* Issues for the Nineties, Vol. 34. Cambridge: Independence.

Warnock, M. (1985) *A Question of Life: the Warnock Report.* Report of the Committee of Enquiry, with two new chapters. London: Blackwell.

9

Hospitals should do the patient no harm[1]

In chapter 6, attention was drawn to the vulnerability of patients. Their vulnerability may in part be caused by their state of health; they may be confused, frightened or too weak to question the decisions of professionals or to ask for an explanation of their condition and its treatment. Their vulnerability may be increased by the attitude of staff towards them and by environmental factors. It is very easy therefore for staff (nurses, doctors and others) to assume mistakenly that the patient does not want to know more and does not want the responsibility of making decisions. Yet worse, professionals may decide that the patient cannot possibly understand.

I am not talking here so much about telling the patient that he or she is dying or that he or she has a chronic debilitating disease which is going to result in a life of increasing dependency and discomfort; I am talking about less dramatic information, such as why a particular X-ray or blood test has been requested, or how the patient's medication will act, and so on.

By not offering patients more information or the chance to be involved in the decision-making process we are doing them an injustice. We are ceasing to treat them as rational human beings. We are reducing their dignity and taking away more independence than does their illness. We are causing the patient harm. True, it may not be a deliberate intention to cause harm – in fact, the intention may be quite the opposite. It is sometimes argued that by telling patients more about their disease and their treatment we might increase their anxiety and thus hinder their recovery. The reverse is probably true. Anxiety is more likely to be increased by uncertainty and relieved by information. Certainly, research has shown that information reduces anxiety and that as a result the patient's experience of pain is also reduced (Hayward 1973). Thus by withholding information from patients we do them harm.

MAINTAINING THE PATIENT'S AUTONOMY AND DIGNITY

During episodes of illness the autonomy of patients should be maintained throughout treatment ... and the active participation of patients in their own treatment should be facilitated by means of open and sensitive communication' (Royal College of Nursing, 1976).

Nurses very clearly share responsibility for all that is done to and for a patient whilst in the care of the Health Service. Such is the nature of modern health care that few if any treatments and their effects can be held to be the responsibility of one discipline. Most treatment prescribed by doctors involve one or more other professional groups. This is probably more the case in institutions than in the community where the administration of the treatment may frequently be undertaken by the patient or a relative. Even in the community, nurses and less frequently other professionals will carry out treatment prescribed by a doctor. It is no justification to claim that I must do something because another professional of my own or another discipline has requested that it be done. In carrying out the treatment I share in the responsibility with the prescriber.

This is true not only of specific therapies but also of the routines of institutions and organized structures. It is very easy for institutional routines to become unnecessarily rigid and to cause a reduction of patients' independence and dignity. In hospitals and similar institutions it is easy for routines to govern all that happens, and even for a routine to become an end rather than a means, so that every decision and every act is undertaken to fit the routine. Patients have to be fitted into the institution and its routines rather than the institution bending to fit the patient. Patients are denied the opportunity of making even the most basic everyday decisions, such as when to get up, when to go to bed, when to eat and so on. The question nurses need to ask themselves is why the patient is being wakened or requested to go to bed at a particular time. Is it because it is necessary to their treatment and recovery? Or is it because that is the time that has been laid down for all patients? If the former is the case, then there is no further debate. If it is the latter, then there is considerable room for discussion. To deprive a person of the opportunity to make such basic decisions as these is greatly to increase their dependence and decrease their autonomy. It is also to treat the patient as a child and therefore to undermine their dignity.

In Chapter 6 I suggested that requiring that patients in hospital wear night clothes had a detrimental effect on communications between them and staff. The wearing of night clothes also restricts their freedom. While it might be socially acceptable for people to walk about the hospital building in their night clothes or maybe even to venture into parts of the hospital grounds, it is most certainly not acceptable for them to leave the immediate environs of the hospital. Thus, a patient admitted for investigations or some form of treatment which does not require that person to be constantly in bed or on the ward is made a prisoner. There may be no medical reason for their not going for a walk or perhaps visiting the local shop. It may actually be necessary for the patient to be physically on the ward only at fairly specified times. Not only is this a restriction of freedom but it may be detrimental to the patient's recovery. A patient who is being rehabilitated might be greatly helped by being 'allowed out'.

It is not only in institutions such as hospitals and nursing homes that this happens but also in other settings. Patients at home may enjoy more freedom than their counterparts in hospital inasmuch as they have control over the way in which they spend most of the day. Even so, the organizational structure of the community health service can restrict the patient's independence as much as a hospital. Because staff are employed to work between certain hours, this may mean that patients have to get up and go to bed at restricted times and that they have to have a bath in the middle of Thursday afternoon rather than early on Monday morning. True, to some extent, some of these restrictions are unavoidable, but we should at least be aware of the ways in which patients' routines are being disturbed and whenever possible try to be flexible and meet their needs.

Generally, rather than insisting that the patient comply with set times, community health workers often refuse to give the patient any idea as to what time of day they will call. The patient is forced to wait around for several hours, perhaps still in night clothes. They cannot go out and do not like to get on with any work in case the nurse calls. They may have to answer the door to tradesmen or entertain visitors while still in night clothes at a time of day when normally one would be fully clothed. Thus patients' life-style may be restricted, and their dignity suffers.

It is one of the first rules of nursing which all nurse trainees learn that at all times they must ensure the patient's privacy when carrying out nursing procedures. This means more than pulling the screens round the patients – that merely allows them to be hidden from sight. To then ask the patient questions of a personal and private nature in a voice clearly audible throughout the ward is totally to negate the purpose of pulling the screens. Since it is the nurse or other health worker who decides when screens are required, patients may find themselves with little or no privacy at times when they would choose it. Take the visit of a patient's wife, for example. The couple may wish to embrace, kiss or simply hold hands, but naturally feel embarrassed at doing so in front of strangers. It is difficult to carry on a normal conversation when you feel you are being watched or when others keep interrupting. Yet seldom in hospitals do patients feel free, nor are they encouraged, to pull the screens round when they have visitors.

It is all too easy, albeit unintentional, for nurses to restrict patients' independence and lower their dignity. To do either or both is to reduce their health prospects. 'In view of this, a fundamental aspect of the nurse's responsibility to the patient can be seen as the maintenance and restoration of personal autonomy' (Royal College of Nursing, 1976). This obviously means that the nurse should involve patients in the decision-making process and keep them fully informed about their nursing care and treatment. It also means that the nurse has a responsibility to question the practices of other health-care professionals and the policies and functioning of the organizational structure if he or she feels they are harmful to the patient or patients. In this context what is harmful is not only the *doing* of harm but *failing* to do what is in the best interests of the patient. The principle of autonomy and relationship to two other principles – *beneficence* (doing good) and non-*maleficence* (not doing harm) – is more fully discussed in Chapter 14.

EXPERIMENTATION ON PATIENTS

Medicine is an experimental science by its nature. Primitive men and ancient healers, trying to treat diseases, must have acted on a trial-and-error basis until an accepted medical practice had developed with respect to the cure of certain illnesses. This history of human experimentation is as old as the history of medicine.

(Varga, 1980)

Much medical experimentation is carried out not on patients but on otherwise healthy persons. Generally (Nazi Germany, it is to be hoped, was an exception), these people volunteer to be subjects of the experiments. Even this does raise some ethical issues.

Take, for example, the Cold Research Unit in England. In this centre the researchers attempted to cause their volunteers to catch a cold in order ultimately to find a cure. This may seem to have posed no moral objection, since the subjects were all volunteers, and the disease which the experimenters were trying to induce was a minor one. Some religious believers might make strong objections, even to what seemed a fairly innocuous experiment, on the grounds that the body is a 'gift from God', a 'temple of the Holy Spirit' and that we have a duty to care for it and not abuse it. Deliberately to set out to abuse the body by inducing infection is therefore wrong.

Veatch and Sollito (1973) list 11 cases of experiments which raise far more disturbing ethical questions. In several of these experiments, large numbers of volunteers were subjected to potentially harmful drugs – in one instance LSD was used – and were not fully informed of the possible long-lasting effects these drugs might have on them.

It was concern about medical experimentation and research that led the World Medical Assembly to draw up a set of guidelines known as the Declaration of Helsinki. This defines the parameters within which researchers may operate, and distinguishes between Non-therapeutic Biomedical Research Involving Human Subjects

(Non-clinical Biomedical Research) and Medical Research Combined with Professional Care (Clinical Research). The former includes research on volunteer healthy persons and patients 'for whom the experimental design is not related to the patient's illness', while the latter involves patients for whom there is a relationship between the experiment and their illness. It is to this category of research that we now turn our attention.

To some extent, of course, any medical treatment is in the nature of an experiment. The patient reports with a set of signs and symptoms. The doctor makes a diagnosis and prescribes treatment, but can never be absolutely certain that the treatment will be successful. The dosage of a drug may need adjusting or it may be necessary to try another form of treatment. The process cannot be likened to the trial-and-error of primitive people, for obviously doctors base their decisions on knowledge gleaned from the work of others and from their own experience. Nevertheless, there is always present an element of the experimental. It is important to acknowledge this before making statements about the rightness or wrongness of experimentation on patients.

Many authorities have traditionally distinguished between two types of experiment: *therapeutic* and *non-therapeutic*. Therapeutic experiments are those designed to benefit the subjects, to find a cure for their disease or alleviate their suffering. Non-therapeutic experiments are designed not to help the research subject directly but to benefit others suffering from the same disease. It has been argued that the distinction is not always so clear cut. Some experiments may benefit the subject even though designed initially to benefit others. For example, experiments carried out on a patient to discover the cause of his or her disease may initially have been designed as part of an ongoing research programme aimed at eventually discovering the cause and then a possible cure. Suppose, by chance, the cause is discovered as a result of these particular experiments and its discovery makes it possible to treat the disease immediately; then the research subject unexpectedly benefits and the experiments could be said, at least retrospectively, to be therapeutic.

To await the outcome of the experiments before deciding their precise nature is, of course, inadequate. The judgement as to whether an experiment is therapeutic or non-therapeutic has to be based on the original intention. If the intention is to benefit the subject directly then the experiment is therapeutic. If the intention is not so, then the experiment is non-therapeutic.

Why, one might ask, is it necessary to make any distinction between types of experiments? Is not the real question about the morality of human experiments? Either it is right or it is wrong to carry out experiments on human subjects. If, for whatever reason, we conclude that it is wrong, then we call into question virtually all medical practice. If we conclude that it is right, then very soon we need to draw up some guidelines and determine some limits. Very soon we begin to ask questions about the purpose of the experiment and whom it will benefit. To draw a distinction on the basis of whom experiments will benefit is a useful one.

If the experiment is designed to benefit the subject, then, having accepted that human experimentation is not intrinsically wrong, it is difficult to argue against it. Of course, other questions do need to be asked about the nature of the experiment, the risks involved and so on but, as a general principle, it is probably acceptable. If, on the other hand, the experiment is designed to benefit others and not the subject, then we are in a very different ball game. To argue that an experiment on a human is justified solely because it will benefit others is to leave the way open for all kinds of obviously immoral acts such as those described in Chapter 2.

We now have to begin to ask a whole range of questions. Will the subject be harmed in any way? Will it cause them pain, discomfort, loss of freedom, loss of dignity? Will it hasten the course of their disease? Is the procedure involved in the experiment unacceptable to the subject? If the answer is 'Yes' to any of these questions, then the experiment cannot be justified, even though it is highly probable that many thousands will benefit. And it can only ever be *highly probable* – never absolutely certain. The reason that it is unjustified is that to do something deliberately which will cause harm to a patient is wrong.

The patient is there because she or he is ill; a patient needs help and care and has placed trust in the professionals. It is the patient's expectation that they will do their best to help and prevent unavoidable suffering. To do otherwise is to betray the patient's trust.

Crucial to all experimentation involving patients, whether it be for their own or others' benefit, is that it is carried out with their consent. That consent has to be freely given and fully informed.

> *In any research on human beings, each potential subject must be adequately informed of the aims, methods, anticipated benefits and potential hazards of the study and the discomfort it may entail. He or she should be informed that he or she is at liberty to abstain from participation in the study and that he or she is free to withdraw his or her consent to participation at any time. The doctor should then obtain the subject's freely given informed consent, preferably in writing.*

(Declaration of Helsinki, 1975)

NURSING RESEARCH

Most research falls into one of three main styles – *experimental, survey or ethnographic.* Some research projects may involve a combination of two or all three styles. Nursing research may utilize any of these three styles. We shall therefore discuss some of the ethical issues associated with each.

Experimental research

So far we have been concerned with the first style of research, and very specifically with carrying out experimental treatments or tests on patients. While some nursing research does involve clinical procedures, much of it appears to have less direct effect upon individual patients. Nevertheless, even though the research experiment may not involve doing anything physical to patients, it does pose ethical questions.

Suppose, for example, that a nurse researcher is concerned to evaluate the application of a particular model to the assessment of need and planning of care. The researcher may want to ascertain whether one model rather than another is a more effective tool in helping nurses to identify and respond to all the patient's needs. He or she may hold the belief that model A is better than model B, where model B is the one currently in use. In order to make the comparison, the nurse researcher would need to have a control group and an experimental group. The nurses caring for the control group would continue to use model B, while those caring for the experimental group would use model A.

This 'experiment' poses several moral questions. Firstly, the patients themselves have no say as to which group they will be allocated. Secondly, if there is already evidence to demonstrate either the inadequacy of model B or the superiority of model A, is it morally justifiable to treat two groups of patients in such different ways? Do they not have the right to expect equality of standards of care? Thirdly, if model A is totally untested, is it morally justifiable to allocate patients to the experimental group without their knowledge? Given that one of the underlying philosophies of most nursing models is that patients should be involved in decision-making about their care, then to enforce a particular model upon them would seem to be morally unjustifiable. To some extent the problem could be overcome by (having obtained the patients' consent to be subjects of the research) allowing them to choose into which group they are placed. However, to do this in many experimental research projects would be to some extent to invalidate the findings.

Survey style of research

This style of research probably poses fewer ethical questions than either of the other two. In whatever way the survey is conducted, whether it be a postal questionnaire or interviewer-completed questionnaires, the respondents have complete freedom as to whether or not to participate. It may be seen as an intrusion of privacy, but the subjects do have the right and opportunity to choose whether or not to allow this intrusion into their privacy.

It may, however, raise questions about confidentiality. It is essential that anonymity be maintained, and that there is no possibility that information obtained can be linked to individuals, groups or institutions, without their full, voluntarily given consent. And, of course if the subjects are patients, former patients or their families, then permission of the local Ethics Committee would be required before undertaking the research.

Ethnographic research

This is a style of research which has been used in nursing. While it may take many forms, it generally involves the researcher being within the situation which is the subject being studied. The researcher may or may not make their presence known, and may or may not make explicit the exact purpose of their research. For example, the researcher may join the team of nurses on a ward in order to observe particular aspects of nursing practice. Now, even if the researcher's presence and purpose is known to the nurses, it almost certainly will not be known to the patients. The researcher will inevitably be privy to confidential information about the patients, which raises one ethical question. They may also be privy to unsafe, or at least less than satisfactory, practice. The nature of the researchers' role requires that they do not intervene, since to do so would invalidate their research.

On the other hand, can a nurse, even in the role of observer, ignore bad practice? The nurse, even as a researcher, is always subject to the Code of Conduct, and therefore cannot be justified in allowing bad practice to continue. The needs of the patients must be paramount and override the need to meet the research requirements.

ORGAN TRANSPLANTATION

In Chapter 3 some of the religious objections to organ transplantation were touched upon. Here, we are not concerned so much with the rights and wrongs of organ transplantation, as with the ethical issues arising out of obtaining consent for transplant, particularly at the time of death. 'The patient's right to respect requires free and fully informed consent from the donor or nearest of kin, as with any other intrusion into the body' (Bandman and Bandman, 1990).

The first issue is that of informed consent. The general principles of informed consent discussed in the next section must apply to the obtaining of consent for organ donation. The person from whom consent is obtained has a right to know exactly what the procedure entails and the purposes for which the organ(s) will be used; that is, is it to save life or to enhance the quality of life of another, or will the organ(s) be placed in a bank for use on a future occasion?

The second, and perhaps more crucial, issue is from whom is consent obtained. We are not concerned here with the requirements of law but with the moral issues. Many people carry Organ Donor cards. This implies that it is their wish that on their death their organs be donated to another. Equally, a patient may make it known to the health workers caring for them that this is their wish. Yet practice is that consent has to be obtained from the relatives at the time of death, and they may decide to override the patient's wishes. This, it seems to me, is morally indefensible. The UKCC (1987) in its elaboration of Clause 9(2) states: 'The death of a patient/client does not absolve the practitioner from this obligation.' The obligation is to prevent release of confidential information. Surely, the same principle ought to apply to respecting the patient's wishes?

One of the problems that arises out of obtaining consent from relatives at the time of death is that they may feel under moral pressure to consent. Therefore it is vitally important that whoever is responsible for obtaining that consent do so in a considerate manner. The nurse in such situations has, perhaps, a role to play as relatives' advocate in ensuring that their rights to considerate care and to give informed consent – and also their interests – are respected.

The nurse also has a part to play in reassuring the patient and relatives that any fears they might have that either the patient's life will be ended prematurely or that they will be kept artificially alive in order to enable the transplant to take place are unfounded.

INFORMED CONSENT

The need for *informed consent* does not apply only to research and organ transplantation but also to all medical and nursing procedures performed on a patient.

> *Every human being of adult years and sound mind has a right to determine what shall be done with his own body; and a surgeon who performs an operation without his patient's consent commits an assault, for which he is liable in damages.*

> (Cardoza, 1914)

And, more recently in the United Kingdom the right of patients to information was spelt out in the Patient's Charter (1991), which states that as a patient you have a right to *be given a clear explanation of any treatment proposed, including any risks and any alternatives, before you decide whether you will agree to treatment.*

The notion that patients have a right to give or withhold consent to treatment, and that in order to make such a decision they have the right to sufficient information, is historically a recent one. One of the underlying reasons is that it will benefit the patient. It has been argued that in some cases being provided with sufficient information in order to give informed consent may not, on balance, benefit the patient. 'Traditionally the Hippocratic physician, in a case like this, who is interested in doing what he thinks will be for the benefit of the patient would apply the doctrine of "therapeutic privilege"' (Veatch, 1981). He would argue that the patient's consent should not be obtained for the patient's own good. 20th-century society has clearly rejected this idea, as evidenced by judgements made in the courts and laws passed by governments.

Having accepted the idea that patients have a right to informed consent, there remain two vital questions. Firstly, what exactly do we understand by informed consent, and, secondly, what of those who are unable to give informed consent?

If the process of obtaining informed consent is to be honest and meaningful, then the patient has to be able to *understand* the information. There is a clear distinction too between *informed consent* and *educated consent.* The former relates to the receiving of information, the latter to understanding the information in order to make a reasoned decision. We shall explore this issue more fully in Chapter 14. Here, I would emphasize one aspect of the information-giving process.

The information has to be given to the patient in language he or she can understand and in sufficient detail for him or her to be able to make an educated decision.

> *If a complication arises after the procedure, patients can deny, and have denied, that they understood what they were signing ... The law says you cannot sign away your rights in advance of a procedure and the courts have upheld awards in the face of signed Informed Consents. You may still be sued.*
>
> (Demy, 1971)

What, then, of those patients who are not capable of giving informed consent?

We still have patients with language problems, the uneducated and the unintelligent, the stolid and the stunned who cannot form an Informed Opinion to give an Informed Consent; we have the belligerent and the panicky who do not listen or comprehend.

(Demy, 1971)

This statement of Demy's has strong paternalistic overtones. The types of patients he cites as being unable to form an informed opinion are probably quite capable of doing so given the information in an appropriate way and the time to assimilate it.

Who really has the language problem – the patient or the professional? Just because someone does not understand or cannot communicate in our language does not mean *they* have a problem. The problem is ours, and we have to find a way to communicate with them. If the patient is 'uneducated' then the professional has a responsibility to educate. To label someone 'unintelligent' is in many instances to make a subjective judgement based on opinion rather than objective facts. The person may be capable of understanding far more than we give them credit, and the onus is on us to provide the information in a way that they can understand. The 'belligerent' and 'panicky' need time, patience and reassurance. Given more information, they may become less belligerent and less panicky.

There are, however, some categories of patients who are genuinely incapable of forming an informed opinion. Perhaps the most obvious is the unconscious patient who requires life-saving surgery. Here, someone other than the patient has to make the decision on behalf of the patient. It may be possible to obtain consent from the patient's relatives but, if they are not available or the situation is an emergency and there is no time for lengthy explanations, then the surgeon is justified in making the decision on the grounds that it is in the best interests of the patient.

A second group is patients suffering severe learning disabilities or brain damage. There have been several instances in which the nature of research carried out on persons with severe learning disabilities has been brought into question, not least those in Nazi Germany. If one starts from the premise that people with learning disabilities are humans and therefore have all the rights that others have by virtue of being human, then it becomes possible to draw up a set of moral guidelines. The two main principles must be (1) to give them the respect due to any human being and (2) to ensure that they are protected from harm.

'If the patient is considered unable to give valid consent it is considered good practice to discuss any proposed treatment with the next of kin' (NHS Management Executive, 1990). The key word here is *discuss*. The doctor does not have to obtain consent from the next of kin, the decision in law rests with him or her.

> *This poses no ethical problem if the treatment can be shown to be in the patient's best interest, and if it is to treat a mental or physical disorder, or it is life-saving. It becomes more of an ethical issue when the treatment is not aimed specifically at improving the client's/patient's health, nor is it life-saving. When it becomes solely a matter of judgement as to whether it is in the person's best interests.*

> (Rumbold, 1991)

In Chapter 15 the issue of autonomy related to people suffering from learning disabilities is further discussed.

A third group of patients from whom it may not be possible to obtain informed consent is, of course, children, and this issue is discussed fully in Chapter 15.

THE RIGHT TO REFUSE TREATMENT

It follows that if patients have the right to informed consent then they have the right to withhold consent. If, having been given sufficient information and having understood what they have been told, they decide not to undergo the treatment, then that is their right.

'Health professionals are not used to having their services refused and are usually shocked when it happens' (Fromer, 1981). One reason for this reaction may be because health professionals, and nurses in particular, work in a hierarchical structure. They are used to receiving and carrying out instructions from above and to giving instructions to, and having them carried out by, those below them. There is also a strong feeling of knowing what is best for the patient who, it is thought, cannot possibly have as much knowledge as the professional. The refusal to consent to treatment is often viewed as a criticism of the professional's competence.

If patients refuse treatment, then this must be seen as a function of their autonomy, and health professionals have a responsibility to find out the reason for refusal. The patient's refusal may be based on accurate information and rationality or it may be based on inaccurate information and emotion. If the former, then the professional should respect that decision but, if the latter, the professional has a responsibility to provide more accurate information. It is vital too to give the patient unlimited opportunity to change his or her mind. The consent form, once signed, is not binding. The patient can request that it be torn up.

The situation may become complicated when the patient is considered mentally unbalanced. Here it may be justifiable to claim that the patient, albeit temporarily, is incapable of making a rational decision either to consent to or to refuse treatment. The professional is then justified in deciding in the best interests of the patient whether or not the treatment should be given. In practice, what frequently happens is that the patient is asked first if he or she will voluntarily assent to treatment. If he or she does, then the professional feels justified in going ahead. If the patient refuses, the professional may then judge him or her to be incompetent and feel justified in giving the treatment without consent. The professional thereby lays himself or herself open to the criticism that voluntary compliance indicates rationality while refusal indicates incompetence. To put it simply: 'If you agree with me you are rational, if you disagree you are not.' The judgement about a patient's competence to choose must be made before giving him or her the choice.

THE RIGHT TO TREATMENT

So far in this chapter we have been concerned with the patient's rights to information and to decide to decline the treatment offered. There is a further aspect which needs to be considered. What if, having been given the information, the patient demands treatment which the health professional considers not to be beneficial, or to us a term now frequently used *futile*?

The principle of patient autonomy as underpinning clinical decision-making has evolved as a means of protecting patients from inappropriate or non-beneficial interventions. It reflects a consensus view that patients' rights should be protected and provides a standard against which health professionals can be judged.

> *Unfortunately, no comparable ethical consensus or body of legal law exists when the issue is not the right of patients to refuse treatment but instead is the limit to their rights to receive treatments. This issue appears when treatments under consideration have little chance to succeed or, on balance, provide little or no advantage to patients compared with the burdens that accompany their implementation. The term medical 'futility' has come to encompass this group of problematic treatments.*

> (Spritz, 1997)

This to some extent 'turns on its head' a commonly held belief that much unnecessary treatment is carried out because, for whatever motives, doctors want to do it. The rise in the patients' rights movement has meant that patients themselves and/or their families might expect treatments which in the considered view of the professional are unwarranted.

Treatments may be considered futile on three grounds. First, that the benefit of the treatment is unlikely to be realized – in other words the chances of a beneficial outcome are small. Second, that the treatment will achieve nothing more than maintaining the *status quo* – as, for example, in the case of Tony Bland referred to in Chapter 7, where continuation of artificial feeding and hydration would have probably only served to continue his existence in a permanent vegetative state. And, third, where the cost-effectiveness of the treatment is debatable and expenditure on it deprives other patients of scarce resources. This third issue is further discussed in Chapter 13.

Here we are concerned with the first two grounds. Suppose a patient having been informed of the consequences, both beneficial and detrimental of a treatment, nevertheless decides that they want the treatment even though in the judgement of the professional the benefits are outweighed by the detrimental outcomes. Take, for example, the case of an 18-year-old youth who is a keen athlete and who requests that he be given anabolic steroids to enhance his performance. He knows the drugs will enhance his performance, he has been fully informed of the detrimental effects on his overall health of taking the drugs, and is also aware that if 'found out' he will face disciplinary action. Having taken all these factors into account he still demands the treatment. In this case the benefits will, in terms of the youth's health, be small. He will increase his level of athletic achievement in the short term, but in the longer term will not increase his overall health status and may actually harm it. The detrimental effects (leaving out the legal consequences) are likely to outweigh the beneficial effects in terms of his health. The doctor then clearly has a right, even a duty, to refuse to prescribe the drugs. The treatment would be *futile*.

To return to the Tony Bland case. In this case, medical opinion was that artificial feeding and hydration was futile in that all it served to do was to maintain the patient in his current state. Suppose then, that the doctors had decided to cease the treatment but the parents had demanded it be continued. Should the parents have had the right to require that the treatment be continued? In this re-writing of the case the continuation (or even initiation) of the treatment is considered *futile* by the professionals, but nevertheless desirable by the family. It has been argued by some (Truog *et al.*, 1992) that patient or surrogate control should not be limited. That if we are to accord patients, or when they are incompetent, their surrogates on their behalf, the right to exercise autonomy, we have no right to deny them that right even on the grounds of futility. However, although, as Spritz (1997) states 'there is always a very strong presumption of patient autonomy, there are clearly instances ... in which patient, professional, or societal considerations reasonably lead to limitations to the absolute right of patient determinism.' In the case under discussion one could equally substitute the patient's surrogate or family for the patient. In other words there are occasions when the health professional is justified in overriding the patient, 'or the patient's family', autonomy.

SUMMARY

In this chapter we have considered some of the ways in which patients' vulnerability may put them at risk of being harmed. Some of the issues considered, such as freedom of choice about getting up, when to eat, what to wear, seem rather undramatic when compared with the issues raised by research, organ transplants and informed consent. They may be less dramatic in their effects, but the moral principles involved are equally important. We are concerned throughout with basic human rights and freedom.

There is no great difference in principle between denying the patient the right to decide what to wear and the right to decide whether to undergo treatment. To deny either is to restrict his or her autonomy. Paternalism means controlling the activities of another, and a health professional may justify a paternalistic action on the grounds that it will benefit the patient. Autonomy and paternalism frequently conflict, especially in the matter of informed consent, and when they do dilemmas arise.

> *Paternalism may be justified, usually when the client's safety is in jeopardy and paternalistic action will prevent harm, but these instances are few and far between. Careful deliberation is necessary before paternalism in informed consent can be justified. Restricting liberty is almost never morally permissible.*

(Fromer, 1981)

We shall return to many of the issues raised in this chapter, and in particular to the relationship between autonomy and paternalistic beneficence, in later chapters.

Issues for Discussion

How much information?
The law in the United Kingdom does not, at present, require doctors to provide patients with all the information about their treatment if it can be shown that withholding some information is in the best interests of the patient.

The leading case is *Sidaway v Board of Governors of Bethlem Royal Hospital* (1985).

CASE

Mrs Sidaway had suffered for some time from recurring pain in her neck, right shoulder and arm. She was operated on by a senior neurosurgeon at the Bethlem Royal Hospital. Even if the operation had been carried out with all due care and skill there was a known risk of 1–2% of damage to the nerve root and spinal column. Although the risk of damage to the spinal column was less than that to the nerve root, the consequences were more severe. Mrs Sidaway suffered that damage and was left severely disabled after the operation. She brought an action in negligence claiming that she had not been given adequate warning of the risks of the operation. It was revealed during the court case that while the surgeon had informed her of the risk of damage to the nerve root he had not told her of the risk of damage to the spinal column. In acting in this way he was conforming to what in 1974 would have been accepted as standard medical practice by a responsible and skilled body of neurosurgeons. The House of Lords rejected the claim that the surgeon had acted negligently. The majority held that the test which a court should use in deciding whether the advice given was negligent was the same as that used in deciding whether medical treatment was negligent – the *Bolam test*. This test provides that a doctor *is not guilty of negligence if he or she has acted in accordance with a practice accepted as proper by a responsible body of medical men.*

In terms of which risks must be disclosed, in *Sidaway* it was suggested that the degree of risk and the seriousness of the consequences if the risk materialized were relevant considerations. Minimal risks – for example a risk of paralysis of less than 1% did not have to be disclosed. However, if the treatment posed a serious risk of a major complication such as a 10% risk of a cerebral vascular accident this must be disclosed to the patient.

What are the ethical issues here? Would the ethical notions of *informed consent* as outlined in this chapter contradict or comply with the legal view as given in *Sidaway*? What are the implications for the nurse? What should a nurse do if he or she disagrees with a doctor's decision not to disclose information about a risk of low degree, i.e. 1–2%, but with very serious consequences should it materialize, e.g. permanent paralysis?

NOTES

1. Florence Nightingale, *Notes on Hospitals,* 1859.
2. This refers to Clause 9 of the 2nd edition of the Code. In the 3rd edition (1992), this clause has been renumbered as Clause 10.

REFERENCES

Bandman, E.L. & Bandman, B. (1990) *Nursing Ethics Through the Life Span,* 2nd edn. Englewood Cliffs, NJ: Prentice-Hall.

Cardoza, B.N. (1914) Schloendorf v New York Hospital. In Gorovitz, S. *et al.* (eds) (1976) *Moral Problems in Medicine.* Englewood Cliffs, NJ: Prentice-Hall.

Declaration of Helsinki, adopted by the 18th World Medical Assembly in 1964 in Helsinki, and revised by the 29th World Medical Assembly in Tokyo, 1975.

Demy, N.J. (1971) Informed Opinion on Informed Consent. In Gorovits, S. *et al.* (eds) (1976) *Moral Problems in Medicine.* Englewood Cliffs, NJ: Prentice-Hall.

Department of Health (1991) *The Patient's Charter.* London: HMSO.

Fromer, M.J. (1981) *Ethical Issues in Health Care.* St Louis: C.V. Mosby.

Hayward, J. (1973) *Information – a Prescription against Pain.* London: RCN.

NHS Management Executive (1990) *A Guide to Consent for Examination or Treatment.* London: NHS Management Executive.

Royal College of Nursing (1976) *RCN Code of Professional Conduct – a Discussion Document.* London: RCN.

Rumbold, G. (1991) *Ethics in Nursing and Midwifery Practice.* London: Distance Learning Centre, South Bank Polytechnic.

Spritz, N. (1997) Physicians and medical futility: experience in the setting of general medical care. In Zucker, M.B. & Zucker, H.D. (eds) *Medical Futility and the Evaluation of Life-sustaining Interventions.* Cambridge: Cambridge University Press.

Truog, R.D. *et al.* (1992) The problem with futility. *New England Journal of Medicine,* 362, 1560–1564.

UKCC (United Kingdom Central Council for Nursing, Midwifery and Health Visiting) (1987) *Confidentiality: an Elaboration of Clause 9 of the Second Edition of the UKCC's Code of Professional Conduct for the Nurse, Midwife and Health Visitor.* London: UKCC.

Varga, A.C. (1980) *The Main Issues in Bioethics.* New York: Paulist Press.

Veatch, R.M. (1981) *A Theory of Medical Ethics.* New York: Basic Books.

Veatch, R.M. & Sollito, S. (1973) *Human Experimentations – the Ethical Questions Persist.* Hasting Centre Report, cited in Varga, A.C. (1980) *The Main Issues in Bioethics.* New York: Paulist Press.

FURTHER READING

Besch, L.B. (1979) Informed consent: a patient's right. *Nursing Outlook*, 27(1), 32–35.

Freedman, B. (1975) A moral theory of informed consent. *Hastings Centre Report*, 5(4), 32–39.

Gorovitz, S. *et al.* (eds) (1976) *Moral Problems in Medicine*. Englewood Cliffs, NJ: Prentice-Hall.
See collections of papers on 'Informed Consent' and 'Paternalism'.

Ramsey, P. (1970) *The Patient as a Person*. New Haven, CT: Yale University Press.

Smith, H.W. (1975) *Strategies of Social Research: the Methodological Imagination*. London: Prentice-Hall.
See Chapter 1: 'Ethical Commitments in Social and Behavioural Research', for a fuller discussion of the issues raised here.

Thompson, I.E. Melia, K.M. & Boyd, K.M. (1983) *Nursing Ethics*. Edinburgh: Churchill Livingstone.
See in particular Chapter 4 on 'Moral Dilemmas in Direct Nurse–Patient Relationships'.

Zucker, M.B. & Zucker, H.D. (eds) (1997) *Medical Futility and the Evaluation of Life-sustaining Interventions*. Cambridge: Cambridge University Press.

10

Confidentiality

Most, if not all, codes of nursing ethics include statements about confidentiality, though none claims that all that passes between patient and nurse shall in all circumstances be regarded as confidential. There seems to be debate as to what information can be regarded as confidential, and whether in certain circumstances confidential information can or should be divulged. We shall explore these issues later, but first we must consider why the notion of confidentiality figures so frequently in nursing codes of ethics.

THE NURSE–PATIENT RELATIONSHIP

The relationship between nurse and patient, as between doctor and patient, is *special*. 'Special relationships are those in which particular duties and obligations are owed and in which certain duties and obligations go beyond the scope of ordinary social intercourse' (Fromer, 1981). That in the nurse–patient relationship 'particular duties and obligations are owed' is a generally accepted idea. Nursing codes set out the duties of nurses toward patients and certainly some of these are beyond the scope of ordinary social intercourse.

What, then, are the elements of the nurse–patient relationship which make it special? Perhaps the most essential element is that if it is to be effective it must be built on trust. 'Hildegard E Peplau's fundamental view of the nurse–patient relationship is one that builds upon the worth and dignity of human beings, the development of trust, problem-solving measures, and collaboration' (Bandman and Bandman, 1990). And as the UKCC points out, 'the focal word in the definitions of "confide", "confidence" or "confidential" is TRUST (UKCC, 1987). The nurse needs to know that patients trust him or her, that they trust the nurse's professional judgement and the nurse's knowledge and skills. At the same time the nurse has to be able to have trust in the patient, to trust that the patient will tell the nurse all that is necessary to deliver the most appropriate nursing care.

The personal information which the patient gives to the nurse to enable professional judgements to be made is information not divulged in the course of normal social interaction. This then is a second element in the nurse–patient relationship which makes it special and which is pertinent to the notion of confidentiality. Furthermore, the nurse is privy to information about the patient of a private or confidential nature obtained from sources other than the patient. The nurse may receive information from the patient's relatives or medical records.

The nurse, then, knows a lot about the patient, which may be known only to himself or herself, the patient and at most one or two others. The nurse obtains that knowledge solely because of the patient's position as patient, and his or her own as nurse and needs it in order to give care. The knowledge is therefore privileged. This then confers on the nurse a duty to keep such information confidential and gives to the patient the right to expect that the nurse will do so. Confidentiality is an integral component of the nurse–patient, or indeed any health professional–client, relationship. 'The nurse–client relationship is built on trust. This relationship could be destroyed and the client's welfare and reputation jeorpardized by injudicious disclosure of information provided in confidence' (American Nurses' Association, 1976).

WHAT INFORMATION

As mentioned earlier, all the major codes of nursing ethics contain a statement about confidentiality. The 1973 Code for Nurses of the International Council of Nurses state that 'The Nurse holds in confidence personal information'. The 1976 American Nurses' Association Code for Nurses states, 'The nurse safeguards the client's right to privacy by judiciously protecting information of a confidential nature' and the 1992 UKCC Code of Professional Conduct for the Nurse, Midwife and Health Visitor holds that 'As a registered nurse, midwife or health visitor … in the exercise of your professional accountability, must: protect all confidential information concerning patients and clients obtained in the course of professional practice and make disclosures only with consent.' It seems implicit in all three of these statements that not all information which the nurse gains is to be held in confidence, that not all the patient tells the nurse is told in confidence, nor is it of a confidential nature.

Some information is clearly confidential, such as information which relates specifically to the patient's condition and nursing care. The patient has every right to expect that the nurse will not pass such information to the patient in the next bed, nor to all the passengers on the bus going home. It may be, of course, essential for the patient's well-being that the nurse pass the information on to a senior nurse or a doctor, in which case he or she should tell the patient so.

> *Where the person to whom that information is given is a nurse, midwife or health visitor the patient/client has a right to believe that this information given in confidence in the expectation that it will be used only for the purposes for which it was given, will not be released to others without the consent of the patient/client.*

(UKCC, 1987)

For example, suppose a patient tells a junior nurse that he or she has been constipated for three days or has a severe headache. If the nurse is going to be able to help the patient with these problems, the nurse has got to pass the information to someone with the authority to prescribe the appropriate treatment. Thus, in some instances information which is of a personal nature may be divulged by the patient to one professional on the understanding that it remains confidential to himself or herself, the first professional, and those other professionals who need that information.

It is not only information which the patient gives the professional that is confidential, but also information given by the professional to the patient. The patient has the right to expect that his or her diagnosis, for example, is confidential information. The patient does not expect that the doctor or nurse will give that information to other patients or the world in general. All information which might be described as 'clinical' is clearly of a confidential nature – the patient's symptoms, diagnosis, treatment and prognosis.

However, some information is clearly not of a confidential nature. Patients will tell nurses things about themselves which they do not expect to be held in confidence, things which would form part of normal social intercourse. Suppose, for example, patient A tells a nurse that he went to Majorca for a holiday last summer, and later in the day patient B tells the same nurse that he is thinking of going to Majorca for his holiday but is not sure if he will like it. Obviously there is no reason why the nurse should not tell patient B that patient A has been there and suggest they get together. To put patients with like interests in touch with one another may well be beneficial to their general well-being and recovery.

Between these two ends of the scale, clinical information and social chit-chat, lie many less clear areas. If a patient 'confides' in a nurse about something in his personal life which is causing him anxiety then the nurse may face something of a dilemma. Firstly, the nurse has to be able to decide whether this information is being told in confidence. If the patient says that it is, that he does not want anyone else to be told, and the nurse agrees to treat it so, then the nurse has placed on himself or herself a moral obligation to keep that information confidential. Of course the patient may not say that the information is to be treated as confidential until after divulging it. This may make the decision more difficult for the nurse. Then again the patient may not verbalize the wish that the information be treated confidentially but may imply it by the tone of voice or other non-verbal cues. The nurse may need to ascertain from the patient just what his or her wishes are in the matter.

What if, for example, the nurse considers that it would be beneficial to the patient for the information to be passed to another member of the health-care team, and for it to be detrimental to the patient's recovery for it not to be? In such a situation the nurse has two possible lines of action: either explaining that it is important to pass the information on and why, and asking the patient's permission to do so, or strongly recommending that the patient do so themselves. If the patient refuses either of these options, does the nurse have a moral duty to keep the confidence?

The response of many readers to that question will probably be, 'It depends'. Depends on what? It depends perhaps on a number of factors: the nature of the information, the extent to which it or the anxiety it is causing may have an effect on the patient's recovery, the patient's diagnosis and prognosis, and so on. I have deliberately refrained from using a specific example because what I am trying to do is to establish a principle. Can we say as a matter of principle that (1) patients have a right to confidentiality, and (2) nurses have a duty to uphold that right?

The question we first have to consider is whether the patient's right to confidentiality is an absolute right. If it is, then the nurse is bound to uphold it. If it is not, then the next question is how binding is the duty of the nurse to keep confidences?

'The patient has the right to expect that all communications and records pertaining to his care should be treated as confidential' (American Hospital Association, 1972). It seems implicit in that statement and the one which precedes it in the Patients' Bill of Rights that there is no expectation that the information is confidential between the patient and one professional but between the patient and several professionals. The preceding statement includes, for example, a reference to case conferences. This supports the suggestion earlier in this chapter that health carers have a right to share information about patients in their care. The patient cannot expect one clinician to keep vital information from another involved in his or her care.

If, for example, a district nurse were to request that a specialist nurse visit a patient to advise on the care of that patient, it would be unreasonable for the patient to expect the nurse not to give some sort of report to the district nurse, in just the same way as a doctor may call in a specialist colleague for a second opinion. In such situations it can be argued that the patient has consented to the sharing of information between two professionals by consenting to see the specialist.

Are there circumstances in which a nurse might be justified in passing confidential information to another without the patient's permission? To answer this question we can refer back to the discussion in Chapter 6 about keeping promises. There we saw that while it might be generally agreed that one has a duty to keep a promise, one could be justified in breaking a promise in order to comply with a higher duty. The same principle applies here. The nurse is justified in breaking a confidence in order to comply with a higher duty, such as the duty to preserve life.

So far we have established two principles. Firstly, that clinical information is of a confidential nature, but may be legitimately shared by members of the health team involved in the patient's care. Secondly, that information, although not strictly clinical, which has a bearing on the patient's progress or recovery may be treated in the same way as clinical information. We now turn to the question of whether members of the health team are ever justified in divulging confidential information to others.

One instance in which clinical information may be divulged is when the law or regulations require it. For example, in the United Kingdom there is a fairly extensive list of notifiable diseases. In such cases the health professional has a duty to divulge the information to the appropriate authority. Beyond this it is much more difficult to make definitive statements.

Anyone who thinks that disclosure of confidential information is morally justified or even mandatory in some circumstances bears a burden of proof. While this approach requires a balancing of conflicting duties, it also establishes a structure of moral reasoning and justification.

(Beauchamp and Childress, 1979)

In other words, one starts from the presumption that confidences should not be revealed and has to produce a strong reasoned case for going against that presumption. This is important, because it means in practice that one's first thought is to maintain confidentiality and only in exceptional circumstances is one prepared to break it. This therefore serves to safeguard the patient's interests and to maintain trust.

Let us consider three quite different cases involving the question of whether or not to break a confidence.

Case 10.1

A married man comes to see his general practitioner. He has previously been to the Sexually Transmitted Disease (STD) Clinic and knows he has contracted non-gonococcal urethritis. He is worried that he may have passed the disease to his wife, but does not want her to know that he has the disease nor how he caught it. He has therefore told the venereologist that he will ask his wife to see their general practitioner rather than visit the STD Clinic. He explains this to the general practitioner and asks him to send a card to his wife requesting that she attend for a routine examination. The doctor, although unhappy about this, eventually agrees because he is concerned that if the wife is infected she should have treatment.

Subsequently the wife calls at the surgery in response to a request that she attend for a routine examination. On examination she is found to have the disease. The doctor gives her a prescription telling her that she has a mild infection which will quickly clear up with a course of antibiotics.

Suppose the wife at this point asks to know what the infection is. The doctor would obviously feel obliged to tell her. Her next question is almost certain to be 'How did I catch it?' If the doctor tells her then he will be divulging confidential information about another patient, information which, in this case, the patient has clearly indicated he does not want to be divulged. Not to tell the wife would be to deceive her and to deny her her right to know. How can the doctor resolve this dilemma?

One way of approaching the problem is to pose the question 'Whose information is it?' In this particular case both husband and wife are patients with the same doctor. The doctor has the same duties towards each of them as he does to all his patients. They each have the same rights. The information, that is the diagnosis and its cause, belongs as much to the wife as to the husband. Since she has the disease the wife has as much right as any patient to know her diagnosis. While the husband might lay claim to a right to confidentiality, he can only reasonably do so when the information is his alone, or when the exercising of that right does not impinge on the rights of another. Thus in this case the doctor would be justified in divulging confidential information, at least by implication, about one patient to another. The doctor does not have to tell the wife that her husband has the disease, nor, should she ask, how her husband caught it; that information she will quickly deduce for herself.

Of course, the doctor should have made absolutely clear to the husband that, in the event of his wife being found to have the disease, should she ask what was wrong with her she would have to be told. One could well claim that regardless of whether she asked for her diagnosis she should be told it – not to inform her of her husband's infidelity, but to prevent her from passing the disease to others.

In certain circumstances doctors and nurses are absolved from keeping clinical information confidential. One example, which has already been mentioned, is where the disease is notifiable. They are morally justified in doing so when required by law or health regulations to disclose information in the interest of public health and safety.

In addition, it can be argued that such acts of disclosure do not involve a breach of confidentiality because, insofar as the relevant laws are public and knowable in advance, the health care provider does not obtain the information in question under the supposition that it will be held in confidence.

(Benjamin and Curtis, 1992)

In the case we have been considering it could be argued that the doctor was justified in divulging the information to the wife about her husband because it is a well-established practice to trace and offer treatment to all sexual contacts of a person with venereal disease.

Case 10.2

Sister Smith is employed as an occupational health nurse by a large engineering firm. One morning, Mr Jones, a fairly senior manager, comes into the surgery. He says that he has been suffering from headaches and dizzy spells on and off for the past two months. On being asked why he has waited until now to seek help, Mr Jones replied that this morning he had 'one of these spells and nearly

Case 10.2 (*contd.*)

blacked out'. This had frightened him and so he had come to the surgery.

Sister Smith asks him several questions about his headaches and dizzy spells, his general health and lifestyle. During their conversation she makes notes on Mr Jones's medical records. She then takes and records his pulse rate and blood-pressure reading. His blood pressure is higher than when it was last recorded during a routine annual medical six months previously. It is also high enough for Sister Smith to be concerned, and she strongly advises Mr Jones to see either his own general practitioner or the firm's visiting medical officer as soon as possible as she thinks he should have treatment. She arranges for Mr Jones to come back to the surgery in two weeks to have his blood pressure checked.

Shortly after Mr Jones has left the surgery, the personnel officer comes in. He knows that Mr Jones has been to the surgery and wants to know why. Sister Smith says she cannot tell him. The personnel officer goes on to explain that the Board will be meeting that afternoon and will be considering offering Mr Jones promotion. What he needs to know is whether Mr Jones is fit enough to undertake a more demanding job.

An initial response to this situation might be to say that the personnel officer has no right to be discussing a senior manager's promotion prospects with the nurse. However, the fact remains that he has, and Sister Smith has to decide how to respond.

What are Sister Smith's options? She could refuse to give any information on the grounds that it was confidential. She could suggest that the correct procedure would be for the Board to require that Mr Jones have a medical examination. She could tell the personnel officer part or all of the truth about Mr Jones's condition.

If she refuses to give any information, neither confirming nor denying that Mr Jones is perfectly fit, then she might in the long run not be acting in the best interests of her patient, for if he were to get the job, the additional stress of his new post might exacerbate his condition. Therefore, she might feel justified in disclosing at least some information about Mr Jones's state of health in his own interests. The compromise option of suggesting that the Board require Mr Jones to have a medical examination is probably the best solution here, particularly if such a course of action is a fairly normal procedure when selecting staff for promotion.

The divulging of confidential information in the interests of the client's own health or safety is generally accepted as being justifiable. In cases of non-accidental injury, for example, there is little or no doubt that the health professional has a moral as well as a legal duty to divulge relevant information. In the case under discussion the circumstances are perhaps less dramatic than non-accidental injury, and the nurses' responsibility less clear cut. In cases of non-accidental injury the health worker has a duty to report relevant information to the appropriate authority. What is Sister Smith's duty? Does she have a duty to uphold her patient's right to confidentiality? Does she have a duty to act always in her patient's best interests? Clearly she does, as do all nurses, and there will be times when, as in the case under discussion, these two duties conflict. What Sister Smith has to decide is which is the superior duty.

Case 10.3

During the course of visiting a patient to give nursing care a district nurse notices that some items of new electrical equipment keep appearing and disappearing from the house. After a while she realizes there is a similarity between this equipment and reports in the local paper of items stolen in the area. When she casually remarks about the equipment to the patient, the patient laughingly replies that it's her son's business. 'He buys and sells – you know, it falls off the backs of lorries!'

The nature of the information here is obviously non-clinical. It could be claimed that it is within the bounds of normal social intercourse and therefore not confidential. On the other hand the nurse is privy to the information as a result of her privileged relationship with the patient. She is in the patient's home solely for professional reasons and as a guest in that home. If she reports her suspicions to the police she might destroy the relationship of trust between herself and the patient. The patient might refuse her entry in future and this could be detrimental to the patient's recovery.

There is no doubt as to her legal responsibility here. If she fails to report her suspicions to the police she could be guilty of withholding information about a criminal offence and possibly be liable to prosecution as an accessory after the fact. The nurse has the same duty as any other citizen to report a criminal offence. Probably the best course of action would be for the nurse to seek legal advice from a solicitor.

SUMMARY

The question of confidentiality is extremely complex, and while the notion of confidentiality is an essential component of the nurse–patient relationship, it is not always easy to decide how far the nurse's duty extends. As we have seen, there are some situations where the information can be clearly classified as confidential while in others the nurse may be justified in breaking a confidence in order to comply with a superior duty. Certainly, some of the most frequently occurring dilemmas faced by nurses are those involving the question of confidentiality. It is perhaps not surprising therefore that codes of nursing ethics contain only rather generalized statements and not hard-and-fast rules. In law, at least in the United Kingdom, the nurse–patient is not privileged as are the lawyer–client or priest–penitent relationships, and nurses can be required in a court of law to divulge information of even the most confidential nature. It is of course still possible for a nurse to refuse to give the information on moral grounds and face the legal consequences of so doing. We shall return to the relationship between legal and moral duties in Chapter. 16

REFERENCES

American Hospital Association (1972) *A Patients' Bill of Rights*, para. 6. American Hospital Association.
American Nurses' Association (1976) *Code for Nurses with Interpretive Statements*.
Bandman, E.L. & Bandman, B. (1990) *Nursing Ethics Through the Life Span*, 2nd edn. Englewood Cliffs, NJ: Prentice-Hall.

Beauchamp, T.L. & Childress, J.F. (1979) *Principles of Biomedical Ethics.* New York: Oxford University Press.

Benjamin, M. & Curtis, J. (1992) *Ethics in Nursing,* 3rd edn. New York: Oxford University Press.

Fromer, M.J. (1981) *Ethical Issues in Health Care.* St Louis: C.V. Mosby.

International Council of Nurses (1973) *Code for Nurses.* Geneva: ICN.

UKCC (United Kingdom Central Council for Nursing, Midwifery and Health Visiting) (1987) *Confidentiality: An Elaboration of Clause 9 of the Second Edition of the UKCC's Code of Conduct for the Nurse, Midwife and Health Visitor.* London: UKCC.

UKCC (1992) *Code of Professional Conduct for the Nurse, Midwife and Health Visitor,* 3rd edn. London: UKCC.

FURTHER READING

Gorovitz, S. *et al.* (eds) (1976) *Moral Problems in Medicine.* Englewood Cliffs, NJ: Prentice-Hall.

See: 'Rights of Privacy in Medical Practice', Cass, L.J. & Curran, W.J.; 'Confidentiality and Privileged Communication', Chayet, N.L.; 'Role of Physician and Breach of Confidence', Davidson, H.A.

Reich, W.T. (ed.) (1980) *Encyclopedia of Bioethics.* New York: Random House.

See especially 'Confidentiality', Winslade, W.J. Veatch, R.M. (1981) A Theory of Medical Ethics. New York: Basic Books.

See in particular Chapters 6 and 7.

11

To tell or not to tell

In Chapter 9 we established that patients have a right to *informed consent* and that if they were to be able to exert this right they required sufficient information. Patients cannot make a well-informed decision about whether or not to consent to treatment unless they are told the truth about their illness, its treatment and the consequences of that treatment. In this chapter our concern is with *truth-telling*, whether doctors and nurses have a duty to tell the truth, or whether there are situations where the truth may be withheld. In cases of terminal illness, to whom should the truth be told, when and by whom? These are questions which are frequently raised by nurses and health workers and these are the questions with which this chapter is concerned.

WHAT IS TRUTH?

Before we can begin to answer the questions posed above we need to establish what we mean by *truth* and *honesty*. Truth and honesty are not the same, although the two concepts are closely related. Truth can be defined as 'the state of being the case: fact' (*Webster's Dictionary*), while honesty is 'fairness and straightforwardness of conduct or adherence to the facts'. Honesty, then, is a dynamic concept; it is about being truthful and is based on one's 'sincere and objective attempt to appraise a total situation and that is limited by his inability to be totally unbiased' (Salzman, 1973). Truth, on the other hand, is determined by the framework within which it is established. It may be scientific truth, as defined by natural laws or factual measurement, or it may be moral truth as determined by God or man. 'Truth is largely defined by how you find it' (Oppenheimer, 1955). In other words, what is true depends on how one sets out to determine it. Hence the debates which have arisen throughout history when scientific investigations have revealed *truths* which have contradicted the *truth* of the Bible.

Being honest or telling the truth means relating the facts as one knows and understands them. In the medical context this might mean that being honest is sometimes to admit to not knowing. For example, when the patient with inoperable carcinoma asks, 'How long have I got?', the truthful answer is probably 'We do not know'. For the truth of the matter, the facts of the case are simply that the patient has a condition which is beyond the scope of medicine to cure and which will almost inevitably cause the patient's death. How long that process will take or whether the patient will die from some other cause in the meantime we do not know. It is important to distinguish between the truth – the facts of the case – and inter-pretation of, or opinion about, the facts. Professional opinion, be it medical, nursing, legal or theological, does not necessarily equate with truth.

TRUTH-TELLING

We now turn to the question of whether one has a duty to tell the truth. In Chapter 2 we saw that in the course of normal social inter-action it is accepted in society that in certain circumstances one need not tell the whole truth. Indeed, it might be preferable not to do so if doing so would cause unnecessary distress. Nevertheless, it is a generally accepted notion that truth-telling is a good thing. Kant, in his essay *On the Supposed Right to Tell Lies from Benevolent Motives*, concludes that 'to be truthful in all declarations is there-fore a sacred unconditional command of reason, and not to be lim-ited by any expediency'. Kant argues that to tell lies is wrong, because to do so always causes injury to another. It is important to note that he concludes that it is in *all declarations* that one should be truthful. In other words, if you say anything it should be truth-ful or honest, but there is not necessarily a compulsion to say any-thing.

How, then, are we to interpret these general ideas in the medical and nursing situation? Obviously, the first point to emerge is that whatever we tell the patient should be the truth. There is no justifi-cation for telling a lie, a deliberate untruth. Do we, though, have the right to withhold information? Or do we have a duty voluntarily to tell the truth, that is, even if the patient does not ask for it? There are two ways of approaching these questions. The first is from the standpoint of the doctor–patient, nurse–patient relationship and the effects that withholding information would have on that relationship. The second is from the standpoint of the patients' rights, in particular their right to information.

Veatch (1981) argues that if it became generally known that doctors and nurses on occasion withheld information from their patients, then the effect this would have on their relationships with patients would be far-reaching. Patients would never know if they had been told the whole truth and would begin to mistrust any information they were given. Thus there would be a breakdown of trust in the patient–professional relationship, and trust is the very basis of that relationship.

If we accept the notion that the patient has a right to information about his diagnosis, treatment and prognosis, then the professional has a duty to give that information. It could further be argued that unless the patient clearly indicates that he does not wish to exert his right to information, then the professional has a clear duty to provide him with it. The onus does not lie on the patient to ask but on the professional to tell.

TRUTH-TELLING IN TERMINAL CARE

'It is an unpleasant task to tell a patient that his illness is terminal. One can understand why many doctors and nurses shirk this duty' (Varga, 1980). If we accept Veatch's argument that to deceive the patient, either by telling an untruth or withholding the truth, is to undermine the professional – lay relationship, then it follows that there can be almost no exceptions to the rule. Even if the facts are that the disease is incurable and will inevitably lead to death, the duty of the professional is to tell the patient, the argument being that if it became generally known that patients were only told relatively good news then they would never know if they had been told the whole truth.

Nevertheless, in practice, patients are not always informed of their prognosis when it is very poor. The defence of not doing so is that such information would only increase anxiety and not benefit the patient. The Patients' Bill of Rights affirms that 'The patient has the right to obtain from his physician complete information concerning his diagnosis, treatment and prognosis in terms the patient can be reasonably expected to understand' (American Hospital Association, 1972). That then would seem to clinch the argument. However, that same clause continues, 'When it is *not medically advisable* to give such information to the patient, the information should be made available to an appropriate person on his behalf' (my italics).

As we saw in Chapter 9, there are situations when, as in the case of a child or a patient with severe learning disability, to refrain from giving information to the patient and give it instead to a parent or near relative is justified. Unfortunately, this clause in the Patients' Bill of Rights is often seen as a let-out. Doctors can argue that it is not medically advisable to tell a patient he or she has a terminal illness because in their view the patient will not be able to take it or that to do so would be damaging to the patient. As a result the patient's family are informed and then the family, with the doctors and nurses, 'begin to play a game with the patient, concealing the truth and offering false hope' (Varga, 1980). This then not only undermines the doctor–patient and nurse–patient relationship, but seriously damages the relationship between the patient and family. The family are forced into a situation of living a lie and may find it increasingly difficult to communicate with the patient at all. The case of Mr Williams (Case 11.1) illustrates this point.

Case 11.1

Mr Williams, aged 72, was admitted to hospital suffering with chest pain and persistent cough. Exploratory surgery was undertaken and he was found to have inoperable carcinoma of the bronchus. The growth was left intact and the chest wall closed. Mr Williams was subsequently discharged home under the impression that when his general health improved he would be re-admitted for further surgery. His wife, however, was told the truth – that he had cancer and no curative treatment was possible. His condition was terminal. After a few weeks his condition slowly deteriorated and he

Case 11.1 (*contd.*)

began to remark that he did not seem to be getting any better, although he said the surgeon had told him he would.

Mrs Williams, afraid that he might ask questions which she would find difficult to answer, spent less and less time with him. She would only go into his room if he called, or to give him his meals and medication, and then would leave as quickly as possible. The couple had been married for over 50 years and had enjoyed a close, loving relationship which was now being destroyed.

One day, Mr Williams asked the district nurse point blank whether he was never going to get better. The nurse asked him what he thought, and then gently confirmed his suspicions that his condition was deteriorating and that there was nothing that could be done to prevent that process. The nurse then informed Mrs Williams of what had transpired and reassured her that her husband had accepted the information. From then on Mrs Williams spent most of her time sitting with Mr Williams and they enjoyed together the time he had left.

Had Mr Williams been told the truth in the first place, then the couple would probably have been spared several weeks of loneliness and anguish.

According to ethical principles everybody has a right to the truth unless they decide that they do not want to be told it. The patient may indicate in some way that they do not want to be told the truth about their illness, in which case the doctor is under no moral obligation to tell them. Unless the patient does so indicate, the doctor's moral responsibility is clear; he or she should inform the patient. 'It seems to me that the physician should not easily assume that truthful information would be harmful to his or her patient. Non-communication could be actually more harmful than the truth' (Varga, 1980). In the case of Mr Williams this was certainly so.

Generally the climate seems to be changing. Oken (1961) found that 91% of physicians who responded to a questionnaire expressed a preference for not telling their patients that they had cancer. A survey carried out by the University of Rochester Medical Centre in

1979 (Varga, 1980) found that 97% of the doctors who responded expressed a preference for truthfully telling patients they had cancer.

WHO DECIDES?

Sometimes when a patient is found to have a terminal illness the doctor will decide not to tell the patient on the grounds that it is not 'medically advisable' or that as the patient has not asked he obviously does not want to know. If the decision is based on the former reason then it is inevitably very subjective. One can never be totally objectively certain what the effects of the information on the patient will be. To support the decision not to tell, doctors will quote cases of patients who having been told have 'given up', whose condition has deteriorated far more rapidly, and for whom death came sooner than expected. The question one has to ask is 'Does that matter?' Is it actually *harmful* to the patient? The patient, having been given the information, has the right to decide how to respond. It is the patient's right to decide to fight the disease, to live to their optimum level to the end, or to give up and let the disease and death take over. To say that this patient should not be told because 'he will not be able to take it' or 'he will lose the will to live' is to be guilty of paternalism.

If the decision not to tell is taken on the grounds that because the patient has not asked he does not want to know, then maybe to do so is on the basis of a false assumption. The reason the patient does not ask may not necessarily be that he does not want to know. It may be that the idea has not entered into his head. Consider, for example, a patient who is still young and relatively fit but has a condition which is going to be rapidly progressive, such as malignant melanoma which is not responding to treatment. If the decision to tell him is delayed until he is very ill, he may be angry that he was not told sooner when he was fit enough to be able to make arrangements for his family and business. He could rightly claim that he had been deceived, because although no one had ever lied to him, nor had he ever asked the right questions, he had not been told the truth. The truth – the facts of the case – had been withheld from him until a time when he was unable to make good use of the information.

Sometimes it will be the patient's family who will decide the patient should not be told. Again, they will claim that they are doing so for the patient's benefit. They do not wish to cause him anxiety or distress or to take away hope. Unfortunately, it is false hope they are preserving, whereas if the patient has the information he can be given true hope: hope of a peaceful, dignified death, hope of living to the end, hope of the next life. While relatives may believe they are acting in the patient's best interests, the real reason for their not wanting to tell the patient may be their own difficulties in coming to terms with death, and fear of not being able to cope with the situation once it is out in the open. In view of their own emotional involvement it is doubtful if relatives are necessarily the best people to make this decision.

Although we as professionals may claim that it is the family who have decided that the patient should not be told, this is not strictly true. At some point the doctor has made the decision to tell the family before telling the patient. It may be that in so doing the doctor is trying to shift the responsibility of deciding on to the family. It may be that he is fairly certain what their decision will be, and by electing to tell them has already elected not to tell the patient.

It should of course be the patient who decides whether to be told. After all, the information is about and belongs to him or her. The patient more than anyone else has a right to it. The responsibility of the professional, doctor or nurse is to try by careful questioning to elicit from the patient just how much, at any point in time, the patient wants to know.

The practice in hospices is to be open and honest with patients. This practice is based not only on the principle that the patient has a right to know but also that their care will be greatly enhanced if they are able to knowingly cooperate in their care. The patient's participation in decisions about their care, particularly in the later stages, is considered to be of benefit not only to the patient themselves but also to others involved in their care. Furthermore, 'the conspiracy of silence around the dying patient deceives nobody except perhaps the conspirators themselves.' (Thompson et al, 1983). It would seem then that a policy of not telling the truth cannot be substantiated on three counts. First, it is wrong because it goes against a fundamental ethical principal. Second, it is seldom beneficial to the patient and may actually cause harm. And, third, it is a futile practice.

WHO SHOULD TELL?

If it were general practice to tell the patients the whole truth about their condition, its treatment and prognosis, then perhaps this question would not need to be asked. The doctor is the person who arrives at the diagnosis and prognosis, and prescribes the treatment. Since the doctor has the facts then it is his or her moral duty to pass them on to the patient. The doctor might, justifiably, decide that in some instances the patient might cope better with the information if it were given to him or her by someone else, someone with whom the patient already had a close, trusting relationship.

The reason the question 'Who should tell?' is so frequently raised is because so often the decision is made initially not to tell or to delay telling until the patient appears ready for it. As a result, several people in addition to the doctor know the facts; the relatives, the nurses, other members of the health-care team all know. The patient is likely at some point to ask any one of them.

Bear in mind that we have already established certain moral principles. One, that truth-telling is good and that to tell an untruth is wrong. Two, that to withhold truth is to deceive just as much as to tell a lie. Three, that nurses as much as doctors have a duty to tell patients the truth in order to maintain the professional – lay relationship and to uphold the fourth principle that patients have a right to information. Therefore, it would seem to follow that whomever the patient asks should answer truthfully, and if they have the relevant information they have a duty to impart it.

In 1985 this author carried out a small survey of a group of experienced district nurses and a group of district nurse students.[1] The survey was designed to find out how nurses thought they should respond to a range of ethical dilemmas involving possible conflict between nurse and doctor. One of the situations with which respondents were presented was this: 'The doctor has explicitly stated that he does not want a terminally ill patient to be told his diagnosis and prognosis. During a routine nursing procedure the patient asks the nurse a direct question about his condition.'

46% of respondents thought the nurse should answer truthfully, while 41.5% thought the nurse should avoid answering the question. The remainder ticked the response 'Don't know' or 'Neither of these'. Almost half of those surveyed thought they should answer truthfully. It would of course be quite wrong to draw any firm conclusions or to generalize on the basis of such a limited survey. What concerns us here is the rightness or wrongness of the two suggested responses in this situation.

Let us consider first the suggestion that the nurse should avoid answering the question. If the nurse were to say 'I don't know' when in fact he or she did know, then the nurse would be telling an untruth and this could subsequently undermine the relationship with the patient. If the nurse tells the patient he or she cannot give an answer and that the patient should ask the doctor, the nurse has effectively given an answer. The patient will almost certainly deduce that there must be something very wrong. The lack of a definite answer may well do the patient more harm than would certain knowledge of the truth.

It is often suggested that when faced with this kind of question the nurse should turn the question back to the patient – 'What do you think?' The assumption is that the patient has already formed some opinion and wants it either confirmed or denied. How the patient responds will give the nurse an indication of the patient's understanding of their condition, and also an indication of their feelings. The problem with this approach is that because it is only used in certain situations it becomes a kind of code, and that in time patients will come to know what it means. Thus, the nurse in using such an approach will have provided an answer which may actually be inaccurate because the patient may assume the worst.

If, on the other hand, the nurse answers the patient's questions truthfully and spends time with the patient, counselling and helping the patient to come to terms with the information, then this may be far more beneficial to the patient. It is very doubtful that a nurse can effectively nurse a terminally ill patient unless there is an openness and sharing of information. One of the main aims in nursing the terminally ill is to help them toward a peaceful and dignified death. The nurse can do little or nothing toward achieving this aim unless the patient is aware of his or her condition.

Thus, it would seem the nurse is morally justified in answering the patient truthfully.

However, either response – to tell the truth or to go along with the doctor's decision not to tell – can be morally defended. The nurse in this situation does face a very real moral dilemma, between on the one hand responding to the patient's right to know, and on the other complying with the doctor's wish to spare the patient anxiety. The UKCC Code of Professional Conduct (1992) states that the nurse shall 'work in a collaborative and co-operative manner with health care professionals and others involved in providing care, and recognise and respect their particular contributions within the care team'. From this it would seem that the nurse has a moral responsibility to comply with the doctor's wishes.

In each given situation the nurse has to decide which course of action will benefit the patient most and cause least harm. Professional codes of ethics, however good, have their limitations. It is impossible to derive a code which will provide explicit answers to every individual situation. 'It is a mistake to think that all a conscientious nurse needs in order to deal with the moral dilemmas that arise in nursing is an adequate code of ethics coupled with a healthy measure of common sense' (Benjamin and Curtis, 1992). At the end of the day the nurse carries personal responsibility for what he or she does and the nurse, not the doctor, nor anyone else, must make the final decision.

Ideally, situations like that which we have been discussing can be avoided. If there were full and open discussion between the members of the caring team then there would be no way in which one member of the team would be able to take a unilateral decision which might subsequently pose a moral dilemma for other members of the team. It is becoming common practice on terminal-care units for the whole caring team, including sometimes the chaplain, to debate and agree jointly whether, when and how the patient should be told. Would this were common practice in all situations!

FURTHER POINTS FOR DISCUSSION

Our concern in this chapter has been with truth-telling and, in the specific area of terminal care, with who should tell the truth to the patient. Since truth-telling is a basic moral principle, then it seems almost obligatory that doctors, nurses and other health workers should always tell patients the truth about their condition. Coupled with this we have the now fairly firmly established principle that patients have a right to information. On the face of it then the answer to the question should patients be told is a firm 'Yes'. However, the dilemma that we face is balancing these two principles against others, such as the duty to prevent harm, pain or anxiety to patients in our care. It may well be that in some situations the truth may actually cause the patient to suffer more pain and anxiety than not knowing it.

It can be argued that in some circumstances the right course of action would be to withhold the truth; for example, when a patient who has had a malignant tumour which has been removed surgically is now making a good recovery. To tell the patient that they had had cancer might well be detrimental to their recovery and in the long term cause them considerable anxiety. In the minds of many lay people cancer is still synonymous with death, and they may not believe that in their case this is not so. True, one can never give a *carte blanche* assurance that it will never return, that there will be no secondary growths, but nevertheless, in many instances it would be true to say that life expectancy following successful treatment of a primary growth was good. Why then, the argument goes, cause the patient a lifetime of unnecessary anxiety and doubt when their health prospects are very good? It is obviously dangerous to try to arrive at a rule to be applied in every situation.

I have in this chapter concentrated on telling the truth in terminal illness. Of course, telling people that they have cancer or are terminally ill are not the only occasions when the truth is hard to tell and hard to hear. Consider the effects on a person of being told that they have multiple sclerosis, rheumatoid arthritis or some other chronic, debilitating disease. Should they be told their diagnosis when still in the early stages of the disease, when their symptoms are relatively minor and causing them little discomfort or inconvenience? I leave it to the reader to explore the possible responses to that question.

Some would argue that the question whether to tell or not to tell becomes redundant when viewed in the context of the nursing process. Inherent in the nursing process is the idea that patients should be involved in their own assessment of needs and planning of care. The nurse, if he or she assesses accurately the patient's needs, should be able to tell when the patient is ready to receive information. In reality, however, the situation is more complex. The nurse may still be under pressure from either the doctor or the patient's relatives not to impart some specific information. The nursing process philosophy merely provides the nurse with moral justification for going against the wishes of doctor or relatives; it does not alter the fact that the nurse still faces a moral dilemma.

We have seen that the nurse, as much as the doctor, has a duty to tell the truth, to uphold the patient's right to information and therefore must alone decide whether to tell or not to tell. Each individual carries personal responsibility for their own moral decisions, and to use as a defence 'someone else told me to' is morally no defence at all. In the next chapter we shall explore further the nurse–doctor relationship and some of the moral dilemmas faced by nurses which might cause conflict within that relationship.

Issues for discussion

John was diagnosed as suffering from myeloid leukaemia at the age of 13. At the time of diagnosis his parents were informed and they requested that John not be told the seriousness of his condition. The medical and nursing staff agreed to comply with their request. Over the subsequent months John was admitted to hospital on several occasions for treatment, and throughout no member of the hospital staff informed him of his diagnosis or prognosis. Two and a half years after the initial diagnosis, John now aged 15 ½ years, was admitted for terminal care. His parents were still adamant that he should not be told the truth about his diagnosis and prognosis. The nursing staff did, however, try to point out to them that John was no longer a child and that if the question of his condition arose it might help him to know the truth.

Three days after admission John asked a nurse if he was going to die, and what it was like to die.

Were the medical and nursing staff justified in complying with the

Issues for discussion (*contd.*)

wishes of John's parents over the period of time?

If not, then who should have told John the truth and at what stage?

NOTES

1. The findings of this survey and their implications are further discussed in Chapter 12.

REFERENCES

American Hospital Association (1972) *A Patients' Bill of Rights.*

Benjamin, M. & Curtis, J. (1992) *Ethics in Nursing,* 3rd edn. New York: Oxford University Press.

Kant, I., translated by Abbott, T.K. (1909) On the supposed right to tell lies from benevolent motives, cited in Veatch, R.M. (1981) *A Theory of Medical Ethics.* New York: Basic Books.

Oken, D. (1961) cited in Varga, A.C. (1980) *The Main Issues in Bioethics.* New York: Paulist Press.

Oppenheimer, J.R. (1955) cited in Salzman, L. (1973) Truth, honesty and the therapeutic process. In Gorovitz, S. *et al.* (eds) (1976) *Moral Problems in Medicine.* Englewood Cliffs, NJ: Prentice-Hall.

Salzman, L. (1973) Truth, honesty and the therapeutic process. In Gorovitz, S *et al.* (eds) (1976) *Moral Problems in Medicine.* Englewood Cliffs, NJ: Prentice-Hall.

Thompson, I.E., Melia, K.M. & Boyd, K.M. (1983) *Nursing Ethics.* Edinburgh: Churchill Livingstone.

Varga, A.C. (1980) *The Main Issues in Bioethics.* New York: Paulist Press.

Veatch, R.M. (1981) *A Theory of Medical Ethics.* New York: Basic Books.

UKCC (United Kingdom Central Council for Nursing, Midwifery and Health Visiting) (1992) *Code of Professional Conduct for the Nurse, Midwife and Health Visitor,* 3rd edn. London: UKCC.

FURTHER READING

Bandman, E.L. & Bandman, B. (1990) *Nursing Ethics Through the Life Span,* 2nd edn. Englewood Cliffs, NJ: Prentice-Hall.

See Chapter 14, which explores a range of ethical issues related to the dying patient.

Gorovitz, S. *et al.* (eds) (1976) *Moral Problems in Medicine.* Englewood Cliffs, NJ: Prentice-Hall.

See in particular papers on 'Truth-Telling', pp. 94ff.

Reich, W.T. (ed.) (1978) *Encyclopedia of Bioethics.* New York: Macmillan and Free Press.

See especially the following articles: 'Truth-telling: Attitudes', Veatch, R.M.; 'Truth-Telling: Ethical Aspects', Bok, S.

Stedeford, A. (1984) *Facing Death.* London: William Heinemann *Medical Books.*

See Chapters 3, 4 and 5.

Summers, R. (1984) Should patients be told more? *Nursing Mirror,* 29 August, 159(7), 16–20.

Thompson, I. (ed.) (1979) *Dilemmas of Dying, a Study in the Ethics of Terminal Care.* Edinburgh: Edinburgh University Press.

Veatch, R.M. (1977) *Case Studies in Medical Ethics.* Cambridge, MA: Harvard University Press.

12

The nurse–doctor relationship

In my estimation obedience is the first law and the very cornerstone of good nursing. And here is the first stumbling block for the beginner. No matter how gifted she may be, she will never become a reliable nurse until she can obey without question. The first and most helpful criticism I ever received from a doctor was when he told me that I was supposed to be simply an intelligent machine for the purpose of carrying out his orders.

(Dock, 1917)

According to Dock, then, a good nurse was one who obeyed the doctor's instructions without question. She did not see the nurse as having even the slightest hint of ethical autonomy. It seems strange to us now that even 70 years ago anyone could suggest that a group of individuals by virtue of their role should be expected totally to abdicate their moral rights and responsibilities. Even the Jesuits, bound by their strict vows of obedience, have never been expected to obey their superior if he or she ordered them to commit a sin.

Surely, then, it is totally unreasonable for a doctor to expect a nurse to obey his or her instructions if these require the nurse to do a morally wrong act. The question of truth-telling, discussed in the previous chapter, is a case in point. A doctor cannot expect a nurse to lie to a patient simply because the doctor has told the nurse to do so. Nevertheless, nearly half the nurses in my sample referred to in Chapter 11 said that they would comply with a doctor's instructions not to tell the truth (Table 12.1), although not actually telling an untruth.

The underlying question to many of the conflicts which arise within the nurse–doctor relationships is 'Should a nurse always

Table 12.1 Telling the truth		
Possible response	**Number**	**Per cent**
The nurse should answer truthfully	19	46
The nurse should avoid answering the question	17	42
Don't know/neither of these	5	12

obey a doctor?' For Dock, and others like her, 60 to 100 years ago, the answer was definitely 'Yes'. Even as late as 1965 we find a revised edition of Morison's *Stepping Stones to Professional Growth* stating that the nurse must follow orders and uphold the physician's professional reputation.

It is not altogether surprising that *obedience* should have become to be seen as an essential attribute of nurses. Historically, at least in Europe, the two major influences on nursing have been the religious orders of the Middle Ages and the army of the 19th century. In both, the idea of unquestioning obedience is paramount. Furthermore, traditionally, nurses have been female and doctors male. This led in the past to the one profession becoming subservient to the other. However, the influence of the feminist movement has done much to redress the balance.

Generally, the climate has changed. Nurses are no longer taught to carry out unquestioningly doctors' instructions. It is now recognized that nurses have professional responsibility for their own actions. 'The nurse assumes responsibility and accountability for individual nursing judgments and actions' (American Nurses' Association, 1976). This transition from a reacting profession carrying out its activities in response to doctors' orders to an independent one has increased rather than decreased the range of ethical dilemmas faced by nurses. All the time that nurses were expected to obey without question the orders of doctors life was relatively simple. Nurses could disclaim responsibility for the results of their actions if they were only doing as they were told. True, they might have experienced some internal personal conflict, but they could justify their actions by saying, 'I don't personally think it is right but I am doing what I am told and as I have no right to question I cannot be held responsible.' Once nurses began to assume or be given responsibility for their own actions then they had to decide themselves whether an action was right or wrong and act accordingly.

The *professionalization* of nursing has meant that nurses are no longer taught that they are, nor do they see themselves as, doctors' handmaids. Nurses have become independent decision-makers, making decisions about the most appropriate nursing intervention in each case. It is not only with respect to nursing care that nurses must take responsibility for their decisions and actions but also with respect to medical directives. In law it is no defence to say that you acted on the instructions of another and disclaim responsibility for your actions. Morally, it is certainly no defence. Morally, both those who give instructions and those who carry them out are equally responsible.

Nevertheless, 'Should nurses always obey doctors?' is still the question at the centre of many conflicts in the nurse–doctor relationship.

CLINICAL JUDGEMENT

One area in which conflict might arise is where the nurse doubts or disagrees with a clinical decision made by a doctor – for example, if the nurse feels that the prescribed treatment might be harmful to the patient. The nurse then has to decide between an obligation to the doctor (to ensure that the prescribed medical treatment is carried out) and an obligation to the patient (to protect the patient from harm). 'Whatever the strength of the historical legacy and the dominating status of medicine, whenever a nurse faces a choice between obligation to a physician and obligation to a client she must recognise that her obligation to a client is primary' (Benjamin and Curtis, 1992).

Suppose a doctor has given a patient a prescription for a drug which the district nurse is to administer. When the nurse arrives at the house the nurse reads the doctor's instructions and is certain that the dosage exceeds the recommended level. Clearly, in this situation the nurse has a duty to check whether the prescribed dosage is within safe limits before administering it. To give it when there is even the slightest doubt would be wrong. If it were an

Table 12.2 Questioning treatment prescribed by a doctor

	Number	Per cent
The nurse suspects that the prescribed dosage of a drug exceeds the recommended level		
The nurse should:		
give the drug and say nothing	0	0
give the drug and then query it	0	0
not give the drug until cleared with the pharmacist	1	2
not give the drug until cleared with the doctor	40	98
don't know/none of these	0	0
Treatment ordered as 'experiment'		
The nurse should;		
carry out the treatment	12	29
refuse to carry out the treatment	15	37
don't know/neither of these	14	34
Giving a placebo		
The nurse should:		
carry out the treatment	28	68
refuse to carry out the treatment	4	10
don't know/neither of these	9	22

Total responses, both groups (n = 41)

excessive dosage and some harm subsequently befell the patient, then the nurse would be as guilty as the doctor of causing harm to the patient. In the survey already referred to, all the respondents said they would not give the drug without first checking the dosage with either the doctor or pharmacist (Table 12. 2).

Let us then take this a stage further. Suppose the nurse queries the dosage with the doctor who, without referring to the literature, gives the nurse an assurance that there is no need to worry. If the nurse still has doubts they should check the information themselves and if they then discover the dosage to be incorrect, should inform the doctor and refuse to administer the drug. If, on the other hand, the nurse takes the doctor's word for it and, trusting in his or her judgement, administers the drug, then the nurse could still be held to share liability if it has an adverse effect on the patient. It could be argued that as a professional person the nurse should not rely on another's assumed knowledge but should have that knowledge personally.

In this type of situation perhaps the best course of action would be for the nurse initially to check the facts before questioning the doctor. By so doing the nurse would be fulfilling the obligation to the patient and, at the same time, reducing the possibility of conflict with the doctor by at least questioning his or her judgment from a firm basis.

Probably few would argue with the notion that the nurse should question the doctor's clinical judgement when it involves the possibility of harm to the patient. In not all situations are the consequences so obviously harmful as in the case of a drug overdose.

Another situation posed in the questionnaire was this: 'The doctor has prescribed a treatment for a patient which the nurse feels is unnecessary; that is, it will not improve the patient's condition. The nurse suspects it has been ordered as either (a) an experiment, or (b) a placebo.'

Respondents were divided in their answers to (a) with 29% ticking the response 'The nurse should carry out the treatment' and 37% the response 'The nurse should refuse to carry out the treatment'. In response to (b), the majority, 68%, thought the nurse should carry out the treatment and 10% that there would be justification in refusing.

The ethics of experimentation on patients were discussed in Chapter 9; there it was established that to carry out experiments on patients which would not benefit them was unethical, and that to do so without their informed consent was wrong. If in this situation the nurse's suspicion is correct (namely, that the treatment ordered is an experiment and that it will not benefit the patient), then the nurse would be acting in the best interests of the patient by refusing to carry out the treatment. Clearly, the nurse should attempt to ascertain if their suspicion is correct before making a decision whether or not to carry out the treatment. While the nurse has doubts, then there would be justification in refusing to carry out the treatment.

The question of giving placebos is a complex one. On the one hand, it is argued that giving a placebo benefits patients inasmuch as it puts their mind at rest and they 'feel better'; on the other hand, it is argued that it is a quite deliberate act of deception. There is little doubt that those who prescribe and administer placebos do so thinking that the patient is being deceived. It may well be that the patient sees through the deception but, nevertheless, the intention to deceive is there. What the nurse has to decide is whether the benefit to the patient is such that it outweighs the act of deception.

In this, as in the majority of moral dilemmas, there is seldom a clear cut, *right* answer. One person may weigh the two sides of the argument and come to the opposite answer to another. The doctor may consider that the benefit to the patient is sufficient to warrant the act of deception. The nurse may not. Moral decisions have to be made by each individual.

The making of that decision highlights one of the distinctions made in Chapter 1 between traditional biomedical ethics and emerging nursing ethics. That is, between the notions of beneficent paternalism and respecting autonomy. As was stated then and elsewhere in this book, the idea that patients should be able to exercise autonomy implies an acceptance of the principle of informed consent.

The justification for giving placebos is that in the judgement of the giver, the act is beneficial to the patient. By definition there is never any suggestion that the placebo is in itself beneficial, merely that it does not cause harm. The beneficial effect is achieved through the deception – that because the patient is given to understand that the effect will be beneficial then they perceive that that is its effect. Were the patient to be informed of the actual nature of the treatment then it would be less likely to have the effect that is claimed, indeed they may actually refuse to accept it. The principles of respecting autonomy and informed consent require that patients be fully informed of the nature and effects of treatment in order to make an informed decision whether or not to accept the treatment. Thus, if these latter two principles are to be complied with, the deceptive use of placebos is unjustified and their use, if open, is likely to be of little value.

Within the context of the nurse–doctor relationship the issues are further compounded by the way in which that relationship is perceived. 'A physician who sees himself as an independent omnipotent man with mystical healing powers relates to co-workers as he does to patients and therefore insists that nurses and other health providers serve him in his so-called "captain of the ship" role' (Kalisch and Kalisch, 1977). The doctor may take the stance 'OK, you may not agree with me, but what I say goes'.

The nurse, in essence, faces a double problem. He or she has first to decide whether or not a particular action, such as giving a placebo, is right; then whether to obey the doctor. Nurses have traditionally obeyed doctors and doctors expect nurses to carry out their orders. In refusing to obey, the nurse is going against the traditional norms of behaviour and also the doctor's expectations.

Obviously there are circumstances in which obedience is necessary. In an emergency situation, such as a cardiac arrest, it is essential that someone assumes control and others respond to his or her orders. Nurses, doctors and other health workers have to be able to react quickly and responsively to orders. This forms an essential part of their training. People who are trained to respond quickly to orders in some situations may find it difficult to do other than obey in other situations.

The doctor is responsible for the medical care and treatment of the patient. He or she is obviously more knowledgeable about medical care than is the nurse. Therefore, it can be argued that nurses should follow doctors' orders because it is reasonable to expect them to be correct, and that the patient is more likely to benefit if the nurse does so than if he or she does not. However, doctors are human and fallible and their judgments can be wrong. If the nurse unquestioningly carries out all medical orders it could result in harm to the patient.

In so far as a nurse has an obligation to follow a doctor's orders it is only a prima facie obligation and may be overridden in certain circumstances by other factors. A nurse must be careful not to confuse a well-grounded prima facie obligation with blind faith.

(Benjamin and Curtis, 1992)

SPECIALIST AND EXTENDED ROLES

There have been two important developments in nursing in recent years: the emergence of the *specialist nurse*, and the *extended role* of the nurse. These expansions of the traditional role of the nurse have increased the likelihood of conflict within the nurse–doctor relationship, and have done so chiefly in two ways.

Firstly, nurses having acquired this expansion of their knowledge and skills feel more able to question the decisions of doctors. Specialist nurses may, quite justifiably, feel that their knowledge in their field is superior to that of a particular doctor. The nurse is working within the speciality – say, terminal care – on a daily basis and dealing almost exclusively with the terminally ill. The doctor, on the other hand, may be new to this work or may only be treating a handful of terminally ill patients amongst a varied case-load. Furthermore, the nurse generally spends more time with each patient than does the doctor and so is in a better position to know the patient's individual needs, preferences, hopes and anxieties. The nurse may indeed be better able than the doctor to judge what is the most appropriate care for the patient.

What, then, if the nurse is firmly of the opinion that the doctor's suggested treatment is not the most appropriate? The first question nurses needs to ask themselves is 'To what extent is the treatment the doctor has ordered *nursing* care and to what extent is it *medical* care?' Clearly, the nurse is better able than the doctor to assess nursing needs and prescribe nursing care. Nurses would be failing in their duty to the patient if they carried out nursing care which they considered either inappropriate or inadequate. Equally clearly, the doctor, rather than the nurse, is better able to assess medical needs and prescribe medical care. The nurse may not agree with the doctor's decisions; he or she might say, 'That is not what I would do', in which case the nurse would be justified in discussing his or her thoughts with the doctor. However, unless the treatment is harmful to the patient, the nurse should, at the end of the day, comply with the doctor's instructions. The nurse, however specialized, is a specialist in nursing in a particular field. The nurse is not a medical specialist. It is extremely important that nurses, as indeed all professionals, should recognize their limitations.

The second area of conflict might arise from role expectation. Doctors, aware that there is something called *the extended role of the nurse* and that nurses can now perform certain tasks formerly considered to be medical, might expect that all nurses can perform those tasks. Doctors may not be aware of (or if they are might think them petty) the regulations governing the extended role of the nurse. In the United Kingdom quite clear regulations exist which make requirements of the nurse, the employing authority and the doctor. The nurse's role can be legally extended in the following circumstances:

1. *The nurse has been specifically and adequately trained for the performance of the new task and she agrees to undertake it.*

2. *This training has been recognised as satisfactory by the employing authority.*

3. *The new task has been recognised by the profession and by the employing authority as a task which may be properly delegated to a nurse.*

4. *The delegating doctor has been assured of the competence of the individual nurse concerned.*

(DHSS, 1977)

If all concerned are fully aware of and comply with the regulations there should, in theory, be no conflict. Nevertheless, conflicts do arise. Consider the situation outlined in Case 12.1.

Case 12.1

Sister Johnson, whilst working for Health Authority A, receives training in, and is given a certificate of competence to perform, venepuncture. She continues in their employment for a few years during which time she frequently carries out this procedure. After three years she moves and takes up employment with Health Authority B. She is not allowed by her new employers to carry out this procedure until she undertakes their training and they are assured of her competence to do the task. This Sister Johnson accepts, although she thinks it a little absurd. After all, her new

Case 12.1 (contd.)

employers are more than happy for her to carry out procedures she learned during her basic training and yet has not practiced for some time.

Dr Phillips, the general practitioner with whom Sister Johnson now works, asks her one day to take a sample of blood from a patient whom she is about to visit. Sister Johnson explains the situation to him. Dr Phillips says, 'Just this once won't matter. I am confident in your ability to do it and you've had plenty of experience. Don't worry, if there is any come-back I will back you up.'

When the nurses in the survey were posed this type of situation 95% ticked the response 'The nurse should refuse to carry out the procedure' (Table 12.3). It might be easy to assume from this result that the situation posed no real dilemma, that the decision to refuse was clear cut. Let us consider the possible consequences, firstly, of refusing to carry out the procedure and, secondly, of agreeing to do so.

Sister Johnson is new to the area; she has recently joined the health-care team and is keen to build good working relationships within the team. She also has ideas that she hopes to implement and for which she will need the cooperation of the general practitioners, including Dr Phillips. In refusing to do 'a favour' for Dr Phillips she may have jeopardized future working relationships. Her refusal might be interpreted as non-cooperation. Her refusal might consequently be detrimental to patient care. So one might conclude

Table 12.3 Conflict arising from extended role

	Number	Per cent
Doctors asks nurse to carry out procedure for which she is not 'certificated' by her employing authority		
The nurse should:		
refuse to carry out the procedure	39	95
agree to carry out procedure	2	5
don't know	0	0

that she could be justified in carrying out the procedure, at least on this one occasion. However, the argument is somewhat conjectural.

What, then, if she were to carry out the procedure? Obviously, if it were discovered by her employer that she had done so she would be liable to disciplinary action. She has obligations to her employer which are both moral and legal. Although in some circumstances it is possible to argue a very strong moral case for breaking the law, in this particular situation it most definitely is not. Suppose, too, that as a result of Sister Johnson's taking this patient's blood the patient is harmed in some way. Suppose he becomes infected, or because Sister Johnson incorrectly handles the specimen the results of the test are invalidated, then whatever Dr Phillips has said about backing her up, she would be personally accountable for the outcome of her actions.

The extended role of the nurse is of course about much more than performing particular *tasks*. Although on the surface the conflict may appear to be about the task, it is underlaid by a difference in interpretation of *role*. Role can be defined in terms of the rights and obligations accorded to the incumbent of a particular position.

Although the DHSS regulations of 1977 at the time of writing still stand, thinking within the professions has moved on. More emphasis now tends to be placed on the individual nurse's right to decide whether she is *competent* to do something rather than on the possession of a certificate. Furthermore, the document itself did acknowledge the rights of the individual professionals involved. The doctor has the right to refuse to delegate, regardless of the agreement of the Health Authority or the nurse's ability to carry out the procedure. Equally, the nurse has the right to decline to accept the delegation. He or she may do so on the grounds of not feeling competent or not having been taught how to carry out the procedure. It would be a professional duty so to refuse as the UKCC Code of Conduct (1992) states that you, the nurse, midwife or health visitor, must 'acknowledge any limitations in your knowledge and competence and decline any duties and responsibilities unless able to perform them in a safe and skilled manner'. He or she may also do so on a specific occasion if, on considering that in giving time to carrying out the delegated task he or she would be putting at risk nursing care to other patients (the nurse may, for example, be alone on the ward at the time).

Many of the conflicts between the nurse and doctor still arise from the doctor's expectation that the nurse is there to do his or her bidding. One district nurse told me that the general practitioners with whom she worked expected her to do all electrocardiograms. They expected the nurse to visit a patient for the sole purpose of performing an ECG. There was no *nursing* reason for her to visit. The conflict here is not about whether or not nurses should perform the task, nor over a difference of opinion as to whether the procedure is necessary, but about the *role* of the nurse. It is about whether the nurse's role is to carry out doctors' orders or to provide expert nursing knowledge and skills.

THE AUTONOMY OF THE NURSE

The role of the nurse has developed in a far more fundamental way than the taking on of previously medical tasks. Over the past two decades the nursing profession has begun to develop a knowledge base which is its own. The re-examination of *what nursing is* has led to the development of a philosophy which in turn has provided that approach to nursing care known as the nursing process. For the first time in its history nursing now has the beginnings of a unique body of knowledge and can therefore define the scope of nursing skills.

Nursing actions are no longer determined solely on the basis of the medical diagnosis but also the nursing diagnosis. Clearly, in planning and giving nursing care the nurse cannot ignore the medical condition of the patient, but that is only one factor among many which the nurse has to take into account.

> *We as nurses make a contribution to the care of the patient which can be quite independent of the doctor. This independent function is well illustrated in the care of the terminally ill patient, who by definition cannot be 'cured' by medical treatment.*

> (Hargreaves, 1979)

The implementation of the nursing process can, and sadly does, lead to conflict between nurse and doctor. For example, the doctor may consider that there is no medical reason for a patient remaining in hospital and order his or her discharge. The nurse may consider that the patient still requires nursing care, and that, until adequate resources can be organized in the patient's home, the patient should continue to be nursed in hospital. The doctor, however, may want the bed for another patient.

Another example is where a doctor 'prescribes' nursing care which the nurse considers inappropriate. It is still all too frequent for a general practitioner to visit a patient at home, and inform the patient that he or she will send the nurse in to bathe his or her, or carry out some other specific nursing task. When the district nurse subsequently visits the patient and assesses his or her needs, the nurse may conclude that the care 'ordered' by the doctor is inappropriate. This can, in the first instance, lead to a difficult situation for the nurse to handle with the patient; it can also lead to conflict between doctor and nurse.

Because of the historical background it can be difficult for nurses to establish their autonomy. Conflict, such as in the examples cited, can arise for one of two main reasons. It can, on the one hand, be because the individual doctor refuses to accept the notion of nursing autonomy, and sees the nursing process as a lot of unnecessary paper work which prevents *his* or *her* nurse from giving *his* or *her* patients the care thought to be needed. On the other hand, and all too frequently, it is because the nurse has either failed to explain fully what the process is, or implements it badly or discourteously.

My own observations, in both the hospital and community settings, are that some nurses still only pay lip service to the nursing process. The documentation is completed, but there is little relationship between the information in the nursing history and care plan and what is actually implemented. Unless nurses show themselves to be committed to the process and implement it fully, doctors are not likely to recognize its worth.

Where the nursing process is being well implemented, doctors recognize its value and respect the opinions and decisions of nurses. One ward sister told me that the doctors on her ward routinely consulted the nursing records and discussed with the nursing staff the nursing needs of the patients before making decisions about the overall care of the patient. Decisions, such as when to discharge a patient, were made jointly.

Conflicts in interpersonal relationships, in most cases, arise from *how* things are said and done. In many cases, conflict related to role perception can be avoided by good communication. If nursing is to progress along the road to professional autonomy, it is reliant on nurses themselves being able to put their case across in an acceptable manner.

DIVIDED LOYALTIES

The sort of situations we have been discussing highlight another source of conflict in the nurse–doctor relationship. Nurses are employees of a Health Authority and through the nursing hierarchy have obligations to their employer. Doctors are employed on a different basis, and they do not work within the sort of hierarchical structure that nurses do. The medical profession operates a 'collegial approach which accepts each doctor as a professional who gives and seeks advice among colleagues, and is open to judgment by his or her peers, but who is not held accountable for his or her day-to-day work to a management hierarchy' (Thompson *et al.*, 1983). The doctor, therefore, has a greater degree of independence than does the nurse. Doctors sometimes find it difficult to understand the pressures nurses experience as a consequence of their employee–employer relationship. Frequently, too, doctors resent what they see as interference by the nursing hierarchy in the care of *their* patients. This can make life more difficult for the individual nurse who feels under a duty to comply with requests and instructions from nurse management and, at the same time, a loyalty towards the doctor alongside whom they work. Nurses may actually find themselves being pulled in several directions; for apart from owing loyalty to the doctor and their nursing hierarchy, they also owe loyalty to the patients and their nursing colleagues.

Whenever conflict arises, nurses must look first at their duty towards the patient, whose needs are paramount. However, that is more easily said than done, for the patient is the one who has the least power. The employing authority, represented by the nursing hierarchy, probably has the most power, for they have the power to instigate formal disciplinary procedures and ultimately to fire the nurse. The doctors' powers lie in the fact that good relationships between nurses and doctors are essential to a high standard of patient care, and to maximizing job satisfaction for the nurse. A breakdown in that relationship can make life unpleasant. Thus nurses work in an unenviable situation which compounds rather than eases their moral decision-making.

PROFESSIONAL LOYALTY

From time to time patients will voice criticisms of the doctor to the nurse. (They may also criticize other nurses or other health workers, and although the discussion here deals specifically with criticisms or complaints about doctors, the principles apply equally to those about other professionals.) If the nurse considers the criticisms or complaint to be unjustified, then clearly he or she experiences no conflict. The nurse can honestly answer the criticism and rise to the defence of the doctor. It is when the nurse feels that the criticism is or might be justified that the dilemma arises. Consider Case 12.2.

Case 12.2

During the course of a visit to a patient to give nursing care, the patient complains to the district nurse about the general practitioner. The patient says that the doctor was rude and appeared indifferent towards her. 'He rushed in here and told me off for calling him out. He didn't seem at all interested in anything I had to say.'

As with so many problem situations, the nurse has first to decide what to do on the spot and subsequently how to follow up the problem.

One possible immediate response would be for the nurse to defend the doctor, saying, for example, that he was probably very busy and did not intentionally give the impression of lack of interest. Alternatively, the nurse could agree with the patient, saying, 'I know he's like that but he is very good clinically', or the nurse could go a stage further and suggest that the patient lodge an official complaint.

In the reality of the situation the nurse's response would probably be largely determined by a knowledge of the particular patient and doctor, and whether this was one of a series of similar complaints or a 'one-off' occurrence. The indications from my survey would tend to suggest that the immediate response of most would be to rise to the defence of the doctor. 93% of respondents ticked the response 'The nurse should defend the doctor', while none thought the nurse should agree with the patient, and the remaining 7% ticked the response 'Don't know/neither of these'. The immediate response to rise to the defence of a professional is probably instinctive and not based on an analysis of the ethics of the situation.

Let us then try to establish a theoretical basis for making decisions about this type of dilemma. Nursing codes place emphasis on protecting the patient from harm and acting in the patient's best interests. For example: 'act, at all times, in such a manner as to: safeguard and promote the interests of individual patients and clients' (UKCC, 1992). 'The nurse acts to safeguard the client and the public when health care and safety are affected by the incompetence, unethical or illegal practice of any person' (American Nurses' Association, 1976); and 'the nurse takes appropriate action to safeguard the individual when his care is endangered by a co-worker or any other person' (International Council of Nurses, 1973). Furthermore, 'The patient has the right to considerate and respectful care' (American Hospital Association, 1972).

From such statements one could argue that the nurse's duty in cases such as that under discussion would be to support the patient. Certainly, if the nurse considered that the doctor's behaviour had been *incompetent* or *unethical* and such as to *endanger the care* of the patient, then the nurse has a duty to act on behalf of the patient. If in this case the patient's account of the doctor's behaviour is true, then the doctor has infringed the patient's right to *respectful care*. The appropriate response of the nurse would therefore be to advise the patient of how to proceed with an official complaint.

On the other hand, one could argue, though rather tenuously, from the same nursing codes that the nurse should defend the doctor and try to dissuade the patient from taking the complaint further. The nurse should 'work in a collaborative and cooperative manner with health care professionals and recognise and respect their particular contributions within the care team' (UKCC, 1992) and 'the nurse sustains a cooperative relationship with co-workers in nursing and other fields' (International Council of Nurses, 1973). Obviously, the nurse should not take at face value patients' criticisms about professional colleagues. The nurse should first try to ascertain the extent to which criticisms and complaints can be substantiated before voicing an opinion, but should remember that nursing duties and responsibilities to the patient are at all time paramount, and those to colleagues secondary.

The nurse, having decided on how to respond to the patient, then has to decide whether and how to follow up the incident. However the nurse decides to respond to the patient, the nurse cannot leave it there, but must follow it up by bringing the complaint to the doctor, or other professional, concerned. This view was supported by the majority in my survey; 75% of those who answered the question said the nurse should subsequently confront the doctor with the complaint, while 17% said they did not know. Whether or not the nurse considers the complaint to be justified, the nurse owes it to the doctor concerned to report to the doctor what the patient has said.

If the complaint is unjustified and the nurse does not bring it to the doctor's attention the patient may voice the complaint to all and sundry, which could be detrimental to the doctor's reputation. At least if the doctor knows about it, it will be possible to try to resolve the situation with the patient. If the complaint is justified then equally the nurse has a duty to inform the doctor of what has transpired, because he or she has a duty to promote high standards of patient care and this must include confronting co-workers when the nurse believes their standards to be less than adequate.

Situations such as that under discussion clearly need to be handled with tact and courtesy. For the nurse to 'take sides' may be unproductive and jeopardize the relationship with either the patient or doctor. It might be appropriate in the first instance for the nurse to explore the situation with the patient, neither defending the doctor nor siding with the patient. The nurse might then tactfully approach the doctor, who might recognize that he or she had been rather abrupt on this occasion and apologize to the patient. However, patients have a right to expect nurses and doctors to be courteous and treat them with respect, and therefore nurses and doctors have a duty to behave in that way. However tired a doctor or nurse may be, however difficult and fraught their previous consultation may have been, or however busy they are, nothing can exempt them from the duty to treat each individual patient with the consideration he or she deserves.

THE NURSE IN GENERAL PRACTICE

Not all nurses are employed by Health Authorities or Trusts. An increasing number of nurses are employed as practice nurses and the employer is the general practitioner (GP). 'Figures now suggest that there are well over 5,000 practice nurses employed throughout the country, and that this number is steadily increasing' (Bolden and Tackle, 1984). The fact that the GP is the nurse's employer brings a further dimension to the nurse–doctor relationship since, within the bounds of the nurse's employment contract, the GP as employer can expect the nurse to carry out his or her instructions.

Many of the problems arise from the fact that the role of the practice nurse has not been clearly defined.

The time has come for the nursing and medical professions to work together to define the role of this professional...Because the development of the practice nurse has been somewhat haphazard, her role and responsibility has not been clearly defined and it is time to do this.

(Bolden and Takle, 1984)

Things have moved on since then with the development of practice-nurse training and education. However, there does still appear to be uncertainty about the role. From discussions I have had with several groups of practice nurses it is apparent that only a few have clearly defined job descriptions. This is a matter of grave concern. It is essential if situations involving professional conflict are to be minimized that the nurse has a properly drawn-up job description. The nurse in agreeing to that job description should ensure that there is nothing within it that is likely to conflict with professional responsibilities as defined in the Code of Conduct.

GP contracts

One of the key factors which has affected the development of the role of the practice nurse has been the implementation of the new GP contracts. It is to some of the ethical issues arising from these contracts to which we now turn our attention.

The Department of Health has set a range of targets in respect chiefly of preventive medicine which GPs have to meet in order to receive payment. How particular GPs respond to these targets can cause ethical problems for the practice nurse.

One GP in an inner city area with a practice population predominantly of social classes four and five (Registrar General's Classification), whose uptake for cervical ctyology was about 30%, told me that there was no point in trying to increase the uptake since he could never achieve the targets. The practice nurse may in such a situation consider that it is unethical in that it is a deliberate decision not to offer a service to the practice population. The question is what should the nurse do about it? Obviously, the nurse should discuss the issue with the GP and try to persuade the doctor to change his or her view. If this has no effect, should the nurse then alone take active steps to encourage more women to attend? Clauses 1 and 2 of the Code of Conduct would suggest that the nurse should do so.

Conversely, other GPs who are enthusiastic to meet their targets may expect the practice nurse to devote so much time to these activities, that the nurse considers this to be detrimental to the nursing care (preventive or treatment) of other patients. How the nurse resolves this situation will depend to a large extent on whether or not the nurse's role has been clearly defined. If it has not, then this would provide a good opportunity for a frank discussion with the GPs about how they all together perceive the nurse's role. If the nurse already has a clearly defined role and job description, then he or she may be in a stronger position to argue that the pressure being applied to devote more time to a particular activity is an obstacle to the fulfilment of that role. In any event, the key issue would be whether or not the nurse could demonstrate that harm was being done to other patients.

Another area in which practice nurses are becoming increasingly involved is the screening of the elderly. GPs are required to undertake regular screening of the over-75-year-olds, and it is appropriate that practice nurses be involved in this. However, many of this age group are unable to visit the surgery and therefore require a home visit. Increasingly, practice nurses are being asked by GPs to carry out home visits, not only to screen the elderly but also to carry out other procedures in the home. It can be argued that in undertaking home visits, particularly to carry out health assessments, the nurse is in violation of Clause 4 of the Code of Conduct. Practice nurses, unless they happen to possess a district nurse or health visitor qualification, are not trained to assess needs or give care in the home. In this as in several other issues, the nurse may find it difficult to take a firm stand given that their relationship with the GP is that of employer–employee.

Administration of medicines

One further area of conflict, which does not arise out of the GP contracts, is that of the administration of medicines. Nurses employed by Health Authorities or Trusts are not allowed in normal situations to administer medicines without a written prescription. However, there does seem to be confusion as to the position of nurses employed by GPs.

> *There are differences of opinion about the question of whether the Royal College of Nursing is correct in interpreting the Medicine Act (1968) to mean 'the prescription must exist first'. Dr Garth Hill of the Medical Defence Union ... stated that in their solicitor's opinion if the patient referred to is a patient of the doctor for whom the nurse is working, then there is nothing illegal in giving a direction to a practice nurse to immunise those patients. Anyone (it need not be a nurse) can administer a medicine under the direction of a doctor.*

(Bolden and Takle, 1984)

However, both the Royal College of Nursing (RCN) (1980) and the UKCC (1986) state that except in emergency situations nurses should not administer medicines without written instruction from a doctor. The administration of medicines on verbal instruction except in emergencies does not satisfy acceptable criteria (UKCC 1986).

SUMMARY

Conflict within the nurse–doctor relationship arises largely because of the way in which that relationship is perceived. The historical legacy of the nurse being subservient to the doctor still influences the way in which many doctors and some nurses perceive the relationship. The results of my survey, though in no way conclusive, would tend to suggest that nurses are prepared to challenge doctors on some issues.

The changing role of the nurse and developments in nurse education have given nurses a greater sense of professional autonomy and greater confidence in their own knowledge base. As a consequence, the chances of conflicts arising between nurses and doctors have increased, and nurses find themselves more often in the position of deciding between acting in obedience to the doctor and acting independently.

Good nursing care is to a large extent dependent on good relationships within the health-care team. In few instances can any one member of the team function without the cooperation of others in the team. Nurses may find themselves faced with the dilemma of either risking conflict for the benefit of one patient, which might be detrimental to working relationships and so adversely affect the care of other patients, or avoiding conflict to the detriment of one patient, but promoting cooperation and possibly enhancing patient care in the long term. In considering a response to this dilemma I refer the reader to earlier discussions, particularly those on *ends* and *means* in Chapter 2 and acting *for the good of the individual or many* in Chapter 5.

Whatever choice a nurse makes, be it in accord with a doctor's orders or in contradiction to them, nurses remain individually accountable for their actions. Nurses cannot say, 'I acted that way because the doctor said so', and leave it at that. They have to be able to justify why they chose to obey, just as much as if they chose not to obey the doctor. The nurse is professionally and morally accountable for his or her own actions.

Issues for discussion

The following incident took place a few years ago and was raised by the nurse concerned as an issue for discussion during an ethics session on a course she was attending.

Staff nurse Brown was working on night duty on a busy medical ward. At the time of the incident the student nurse was on her meal-break and nurse Brown was alone on the ward. An elderly diabetic patient had been admitted as an emergency earlier in the day having suffered a hyperglycaemic attack. Nurse Brown observed that the patient was again becoming hyperglycaemic and called the House Officer. The House Officer arrived and having examined the patient prescribed an immediate injection of insulin. Nurse Brown was called to another patient and whilst attending to them the House Officer drew up the insulin. She then asked Nurse Brown to check it. Nurse Brown pointed out to the doctor that she had miscalculated the dose – it was in fact 10 times the dose she had prescribed. The doctor replied that she had drawn up the correct amount, and said, 'I know what I'm doing, how dare you question my judgement.' She then proceeded towards the patient with the syringe intending to administer the injection.

What should nurse Brown have done, (a) in the immediate situation, and (b) subsequently? What are the likely consequences of her choices of action in the immediate and long term?

REFERENCES

American Hospital Association (1972) *A Patients' Bill of Rights.*

American Nurses' Association (1976) *Code for Nurses.*

Benjamin, M. & Curtis, J. (1992) *Ethics in Nursing,* 3rd edn. New York: Oxford University Press.

Bolden, K.J. & Takle, B.A. (1984) *Practice Nurse Handbook.* Oxford: Blackwell Scientific Publications.

DHSS (1977) The extending role of the clinical nurse – legal implications and training requirements', HC (77) 22, cited in Young, A.P. (1981) *Legal Problems in Nursing Practice.* London: Harper & Row.

Dock, S. (1917) The relation of the nurse to the doctor and the doctor to the nurse. *American Journal of Nursing,* 17, 394, cited in Benjamin, M. & Curtis, J. (1981) *Ethics in Nursing.* New York: Oxford University Press.

Hargreaves, I. (1979) Theoretical consideration. In Kratz, C. (ed.), *The Nursing Process.* London: Baillière Tindall.

International Council of Nurses (1973) *Code for Nurses.* Geneva: ICN.

Kalisch, B. & Kalisch, P. (1977) An analysis of the sources of physician–nurse conflict, cited in Benjamin, M. & Curtis, J. (1981) *Ethics in Nursing.* New York: Oxford University Press.

RCN (Royal College of Nursing) (1980) *Drug Administration – a Nursing Responsibility.* London: RCN.

Thompson, I.E., Melia, K.M. & Boyd, K.M. (1983) *Nursing Ethics.* Edinburgh: Churchill Livingstone.

UKCC (United Kingdom Central Council for Nursing, Midwifery and Health Visiting) (1986) *Administration of Medicines; a UKCC Advisory Paper.* London: UKCC.

UKCC (1992) *Code of Professional Conduct for the Nurse, Midwife, and Health Visitor,* 3rd edn. London: UKCC.

FURTHER READING

Chaska, N.L. (ed.) (1978) *The Nursing Profession: Views Through the Mist.* New York: McGraw-Hill.

See especially 'Nurse–Physician Relationships: Problems and Solutions', Hoekelman, R.A., pp. 330–335.

Beardshaw, V. (1992) *Conscientious Objectors at Work.* London: Social Audit.

Benjamin, M. & Curtis, J. (1992) *Ethics in Nursing,* 3rd edn. New York: Oxford University Press.

See in particular Chapter 4 on 'Recurring Ethical Issues in Nurse–Physician Relationships'.

Lawrence, J. & Crisham, P. (1984) Making a choice. *Nursing Times,* 18 July, 57–58.

Lawrence, J. & Crisham, P. (1984) A study in resolutions. *Nursing Times,* 25 July, 53–55.

13

Is it fair?

Is it fair that one patient should get a heart transplant costing thousands of pounds, while hundreds have to wait for hip replacements? Is it fair that health care resources in one part of the country should be better than those elsewhere? These, and similar questions, are frequently voiced, not just by members of the health care professions but by the public at large. We feel that there ought to be a fairness about health care provision and receipt; that there should be available to every individual an equal portion; and that all should be able to receive what they need. It is with the question of fairness – or, more specifically, justice – that we shall be concerned in this chapter: justice in health care.

JUSTICE

Before we can begin to discuss justice in health care, we need to be clear about what is meant by justice. The question 'What is justice?' is one to which it is not possible to give a definitive answer. The word *justice* is used in a variety of different ways, all of which are legitimate, and can lay claim to being the true meaning of the word. However, it is possible to identify the principal meanings of the concept of justice: first, the concept of justice as retribution or punishment; and second, the concept of justice as fairness, and in particular fair distribution.

The first notion, that of justice as retribution or punishment, is of more relevance to discussions about law than health. For it is concerned with the idea that those who do wrong should be brought to justice. The wrongdoing, and therefore the retribution, may be defined by man or God. That is to say that the wrongdoing may be offence against a man-made law – and called a crime – punishable by society through the judiciary system. Or it may be an offence against the laws of God – and called a sin – which brings about divine retribution. The punishment or retribution is seen as 'just', because it aims to put right the wrong that has been done, or cause the wrongdoer to pay the price for the wrong he or she has done to another or others. Another or others may be a fellow human being, God or the State.

This notion of justice has little to do with health care, though there have been, and probably still are, examples of health care workers using their 'power' to punish those whom they believe to have done wrong. Think of the way in which, in the past, people who had attempted suicide were treated, particularly in general hospitals. Frequently, they were isolated in side wards or single rooms, where they were ignored by the staff. There was the feeling, not openly expressed but nevertheless real, that these people had done wrong (and remember that at one time suicide was not only a 'sin', but also against the law), and therefore ought to pay the price in some way. Also, there was the feeling that through their deliberate act they were causing unnecessary work for the hospital staff, who, after all, had enough to do looking after the legitimate sick. Again, and the author has been witness to this, ECT was often administered as a punishment rather than for genuine therapeutic reasons. In such cases it was frequently administered without anaesthesia.

These are rather dramatic examples. But nurses, and others involved in health care, can and do use other more subtle ways of 'punishing' patients whom they consider to be 'wrongdoers' – not wrongdoers in the sense of being criminals or sinners, but in the sense of being awkward, or not complying with the rules of behaviour. Several examples are to be found in Stockwell's (1972) research monograph, *The Unpopular Patient*. So while the idea of justice as punishment might be of minor significance in health care, we should not totally ignore it.

The second major idea related to justice is that of justice as fairness. It is this idea of justice which is of chief concern here. It is sometimes described as the justice of distribution – that is, the justice (or fairness) of the distribution of some commodity to each individual in equal portions. Seedhouse (1988) suggests that there are three versions of justice as fairness: 'to each according to his rights, to each according to what he deserves, and to each according to his need'.

One interpretation of 'to each according to his rights' is that it implies some sort of contract. If I do something for you, then I can expect something in return. An employer undertakes to give someone a job and to pay his wages; in return the employer has a right to expect a fair day's work. If we apply this idea to health care, then we might argue that there is a contractual arrangement between the health care professional and the patient or client; that, when a person seeks health care he or she enters into a contract with the doctor (or other health worker) and becomes a patient. The doctor, having agreed to 'take on' the patient, offers to treat them. It could then be argued that, in return for the promise to treat, the doctor has a right to expect the patient's compliance.

Does the patient also have rights under the contract? In the employer–employee contract both partners have rights, because both have something to offer the other for which they can claim a right to something in return. The employee offers to do the work, and if he does it can claim the right to a fair day's pay in return. What does the patient have to offer the doctor to earn something in return? In the private health care sector it is payment. The patient can be seen as the employer or purchaser. In a State-run health care system it could be argued that the patient is paying, through taxation or National Insurance, and, therefore, has a right to expect a return for this money. The contract, then, is not with the individual health care worker, but with the health service.

The weakness of this argument is, of course, that not all pay the same amount. Some pay more through private insurance. Do they have more rights to health care than others? What happens if, for example, you contract a chronic debilitating condition, and not only cease to pay into the system – through taxation – but could also be seen to have had your fair share of health care? Do you then have no further rights to health care?

However, there is a wider, and more significant, interpretation of the notion 'to each according to his rights'. It is derived from the idea that fairness is about equality. The notion then comes to mean that each individual has equal rights; that we all have the same rights to health care. If the idea 'to each according to his rights' is not interpreted in this way, but is seen purely in contractual terms, then there are basic, built-in injustices.

However, equal rights do not automatically give rise to equal returns. As Seedhouse (1988) points out, in this country all have a *right* to own their own home. Yet, not all do, because some cannot afford to do so. And, even among those who are able to exert their right, there is no equality about the type of housing they are able to own. To say, therefore, that justice in health care is about equal rights to it will not automatically ensure equality of distribution.

What, then, of the notion *to each according to what he deserves?* This implies the idea that health care (or whatever is under discussion) has to be earned. It is the notion which lies behind everyday sayings such as, 'You get out of this life what you put in', or 'You make your own bed and lie in it', or 'He who pays the piper calls the tune'.

In some areas of life, this idea seems fair and just. After all, if a person works hard, then he or she deserves to receive more. If someone puts a lot of themselves and their resources into forming a business, then they deserve to be successful. If someone doesn't bother, doesn't put in much effort, then they deserve to get little in return. There seems to be some justice in this, inasmuch as it is about receiving one's just reward.

Now, that may be fine when it comes to, for example, the acquisition of material rewards. Can the same be said of benefiting from health care, though? If we accept the idea that everyone has a natural right to health care, then should not the right be independent of ability, labour or wealth? Certainly, we probably feel uncomfortable with the idea that power, success or money should entitle a person to more or better health care than others – especially given that most of those who lack these attributes do so through no fault of their own.

On the other hand, it can be argued that those who have the ability and means to enhance their health, but fail to do so from choice, lose some of their rights to health care. Should the person who chooses an unhealthy life style be entitled to receive the same health care as someone who makes every effort to maintain their health? There are those who would argue that, for example, a smoker who contracts cancer of the lung should not automatically expect to receive all possible treatment. They have brought the condition upon themselves in full knowledge of the probable consequences of their actions.

There are two fundamental problems here. First, where do you stop? Do you refuse to treat the careless driver injured in a road accident, or the attempted suicide, or the woman who haemorrhages following an illegal abortion? The list could be endless, especially in this age, when most of the major causes of mortality in Western society can be attributed, at least in part, to the individual's behaviour. Second, while there might be an overwhelming statistical probability that a smoker's lung cancer is due to his smoking, there is always the slim chance that it might be coincidental. One could run the risk that accompanies the use of capital punishment: sometime, somewhere, an innocent person will be hanged.

So we can see that, although the ideas of justice as 'to each according to his rights' and 'to each according to what he deserves' may have some applicability to health care, they do not seem totally to meet an ideal notion of fairness in health care. What, then, of the third idea: 'to each according to his needs'? Is this more likely to provide a firmer basis for assessing fairness in the distribution of health care?

One of the principles underlying the founding of the National Health Service was 'from each according to his means, to each according to his needs' – in other words, that each individual should contribute financially to it according to ability, through either National Insurance or taxation; and that, regardless of how much, or how little, the contribution, that individual should receive what he or she needs.

On an individual basis, this is probably what each health-care worker – nurse, midwife or whoever – aims to do for each individual patient or client. Not only do they aim to do it, but they would claim that, within their capabilities, they do so. On a larger scale, it is clearly not achieved. The chief reason for this is that the resources available are inadequate to meet the total needs of everybody. Now, if the cake is small, everybody should receive a smaller but equal slice. In practice, as numerous reports have shown (for example, *the Black Report* in 1982 and *The Health Divide* in 1987, republished by Townsend *et al.*, (1990)), there are inequalities in health care. Some receive all they need, while others receive less than they need.

The explanations for these inequalities are in part sociological, economic and psychological, but also, in part, ethical. Some of the inequalities arise from the fact that there is injustice in the distribution of health care. Injustice, or unfairness, in the distribution of health care occurs at all levels, from national down to individual practitioner–client level. It is to a closer examination of the degree of fairness of distribution at various levels that we now turn.

CUTTING UP THE NATIONAL CAKE

We are frequently told that resources are limited but demand is limitless. Therefore, it is unrealistic to expect that all demands can or will be met in full. If we begin from this position, then it is inevitable that there will be some injustice – inevitable, because it means that the needs of some will not be met, while the needs of others are met. Both demand and need fluctuate. They fluctuate from one individual to another, from one moment in time to another, and from one place to another.

In education, it would be possible to ensure that all receive equal shares of the national cake. We know how many children there are, and we know that each of these children requires schooling from age 5 to 16 years. We can therefore divide the cake so that each child receives the same amount of schooling with equal amounts of resourcing. It is possible, although in practice it does not happen. Even if it did, it still would not necessarily be just. For some children this fairly apportioned slice of the cake might be more than sufficient to meet their needs, but for others it might be insufficient.

If simply distributing resources equally per capita is not likely to achieve a just result in education, it certainly will not do so in health care. Suppose, for example, the population was 50 million, and that the budget allocation for health care in any one year was £12.5 million. Would allowing each individual £250,000 worth of health care ensure equality? It would ensure equality, only in the sense that each individual could claim a right to an equal amount of health care. However, it would not ensure justice, if justice means to each according to his or her needs. For it would mean that some would not get all they need – they might use up their £250,000 worth of health care and still be in need, while others might need a considerably smaller amount, even none at all. These people would be receiving all that they need, while the others would receive less than they need. There would also be the question of what happens to that portion of allocated health care which some individuals do not use? Are they to be allowed to, as it were, save it up for when they do need it? Or is it to be redistributed, and if so, when? Clearly, to try to allocate health care resources equally on a per capita basis is not only impracticable, but is also unfair.

What, though, if resources are allocated on the basis of need, so that those with the greatest need receive more? Will allocating more resources to those areas of the country, or groups within the population, with greater need necessarily ensure justice? It will, but only if the total available resource is sufficient to meet all needs. If not, then one of two things happens. Either there has to be some sort of rationing, similar to that described above, or the allocation to each group sufficient to meet a percentage of their needs. Now, it could be argued that if everyone has 75% of their needs met, that is fairer than some having 100% met while others only have 50% met. It is fair only in that everyone suffers the same amount of deprivation. But, is it just? Clearly not, if justice in health care is to be based on the principle of to each according to his or her needs. For what this principle implies is that everyone should have 100% of their needs met.

Of course, what happens in practice is that even though some attempt is made to allocate resources on the basis of comparative need – that is the intention of, for example, the Resource Allocation Working Party (RAWP)[1] – they are then distributed on a first come, first served basis. Then, once the resources are used up, the rest have to wait until further resources are made available.

What becomes apparent from the foregoing discussion is that injustice in health care is inevitable if resourcing is insufficient to meet all needs. There are bound to be winners and losers. Now, given that a multitude of factors mean that, in reality, resources are likely never to be sufficient to meet need, what measures can be used to bring about the most just distribution of those resources?

ARE QALYS THE ANSWER?

QALYs (Quality Adjusted Life Years) are used as a measure for apportioning health care at both macro and micro levels. QALYs provide, it is claimed, a means of measuring the relative value of one health state over another. As a measure, it brings together changes in survival, morbidity and quality of life. It provides a way of comparing the cost, not just in financial terms, of quite distinctly different procedures and/or health problems.

How do they work? According to Williams (1985):

> The essence of a QALY is that it takes a year of healthy life expectancy to be worth 1, but regards a year of unhealthy life experience as worth less than 1. Its precise value is less the worse the quality of life of the unhealthy person.

It is sometimes referred to as the healthy–death scale, because death has the score of zero. A QALY aims to assess the difference in quality of life between individuals. The first weakness of QALYs is that only a limited number of criteria are used to measure quality of life. The second is that it is possible for an individual to attain a negative score; that is, to be worse than dead.

Those criticisms apart, would the allocation of health care resources on the basis of QALYs be just? The idea is that those who score high should receive priority, and, of course, the cost of treating them will be less than those with lower scores. In other words, those who are less debilitated, have a greater chance of survival and whose future life is likely to be of a 'better quality' should receive priority in the allocation of resources. There seems a certain illogicality in this, for what in effect is being said is that the less ill you are, the greater your entitlement to health care.

Perhaps, though, the greatest criticism of the case put forward by those who advocate the use of QALYs is that pointed out by Seedhouse (1988): 'They fail to notice the important distinction between the "quality" of life and the "value" of life.' The use of QALYs as a means of deciding who receives treatment, whether on a national basis, or an individual one, will not ensure justice. For implicit in the underlying assumptions is the idea that some lives are of less value than others. As a consequence, some people are afforded less respect as persons than others. QALYs might provide a useful tool to measure comparative costs of care and treatment, and thus to decide which individuals or groups need more spent on them. What they cannot, and should not, be used for is as a means of determining people's worth. If they are, then the result will not be fair or just.

For the most part, we have so far been concerned with justice on a national or macro scale. We turn now to the question of justice at the micro level, the level at which individual practitioners make decisions. Individual practitioners, be they doctors, nurses, midwives or any other health professionals, make decisions daily which involve the concept of justice. The decisions may be between one patient or client and another, or about how to treat a particular individual.

In many ways the decisions which an individual practitioner makes when deciding between the comparative needs of two or more patients or clients mirror those made at the macro level. On what basis, for example, does a district nurse decide to spend more time with a particular patient, knowing that as a consequence other patients may receive less time than they want or need? Is the dying patient more deserving of the nurse's time than a person who has just been informed that they are suffering from multiple sclerosis? Are the needs of a bedridden patient calling out for a bedpan greater than those of a patient who desperately wants to talk about her impending mastectomy?

In essence, the problem which faces the individual practitioner is the same as that which faces a government or Health Authority. They have insufficient resources to meet either demand or need. The individual, as much as the government, has to prioritize. In many ways, the dilemma is easier to resolve at an individual level than at a national one. A doctor, for example, will elect to treat as a priority a patient whose life is threatened over one whose condition, although serious, is not life-threatening. In the example mentioned above, the nurse would be justified in attending to the patient who needs a bedpan prior to the patient wanting to discuss her fears about a mastectomy, although, in many ways, the latter is a more serious problem.

In effect, what determines choice is immediacy of need. The

needs of a patient whose condition is life-threatening are more acute than those of a patient with a non-life-threatening condition. Equally, the need of a patient for a bedpan is more immediate than the need of the patient who wants to discuss her anxieties. But, of course, not all choices are as straightforward as these. Frequently, practitioners have to share their resources among several patients the immediacy of whose needs is more or less equal.

Clearly, no nurse, midwife or doctor can achieve the impossible. They cannot split themselves in two. In many ways it is easier for the nurse working in the community or for the doctor, because for the most part they have only one patient or client in front of them at a time. They may know that there are others to follow, but they are not often faced with the necessity of having to decide between patients in their presence. The nurse or midwife in a hospital ward may frequently face a situation in which two or more patients or clients are calling for their attention simultaneously. There is, of course, no *right* answer to this dilemma. Whatever action the nurse or midwife takes there will be unfairness. One patient will receive justice while others will not.

CAN JUSTICE BE ACHIEVED?

It would seem, from the foregoing discussion, that justice in the distribution of health care, whether at a macro or micro level, can seldom be achieved. It cannot be achieved unless resources are unlimited. In fact, they would need to be excessive to probable demand in order to ensure that absolute justice was achieved.

To *ensure* distributive justice at the macro level would mean that there would need to be made available, for example, sufficient resources to provide care for the entire 'at-risk' population of a disease or condition should they all require treatment at the same time. On a micro level, it would mean that, for example, the staffing on a ward would need to be such that, should every patient call for a bedpan at the same time, they would all be able to receive one. Such over-provision of resources would in itself be unjust, because, even if it could be achieved without depriving other necessary services, it would mean that we would all be paying more than we need.

However, the impossibility of the absolute does not justify the minimum. There must be a compromise solution. The compromise is to base resourcing on known demand. Known demand can be measured, and the resources needed to meet that demand can be calculated. At a macro level, we know what percentage of the at-risk population for a given condition actually contract it. We know, for example, what percentage of the elderly require hip replacements. We can calculate the resources required to meet that need. Therefore, if we provide that level of resources, we can achieve a reasonable degree of justice. Similarly, at a micro level we can calculate both the probable demands, and the resources needed to meet them, of a 35-bedded medical ward. Thus, justice in the distribution of health care is a possibility given adequate resourcing.

JUSTICE AND THE INDIVIDUAL

So far we have been concerned with justice or fairness between groups or individuals. We turn now to another equally important aspect. That is the notion of justice or fairness in the one-to-one, professional–client situation. The question we are now concerned with is, 'How can we treat an individual patient/client fairly?' 'Justice has another side to it, concerned with treating individuals rightly in the light of their own wants, needs and merits' (Downie and Calman, 1987).

If we accept that truth-telling is a moral principle, then to not tell the truth to someone is to treat them immorally or unjustly. Therefore, to be dishonest with, deceive or withhold the truth from a patient is unjust. Equally, to disallow a patient or client autonomy, to fail to involve them in decision-making about their care, is to treat them unjustly. For it is to not respect them as persons. Justice in our dealings with others arises out of the supreme principle of respect for them as persons. This applies not only in health care but also in our dealings with others generally.

JUSTICE AND MEDICAL FUTILITY

In Chapter 9 the concept of medical futility was discussed in terms of the use of treatments which might be of little or no immediate benefit to the patient concerned. Another reason for denying a patient a particular treatment may be 'because its cost is disproportionate to its benefits, it deprives other patients of scarce resources, or it conflicts with broader societal values.' (Spritz, 1997).

While it is important to distinguish between decisions made to withhold treatment on the basis of futility and those based on rationing, there is often an overlap between the two and the distinction may be ambiguous. In the real world, where resources are limited, it is not possible to base decisions as to whether or not to give a particular treatment solely on individual needs and possible benefits. The notion of medical futility can provide a useful criterion for deciding to whom resources should be allocated. For example, if a costly treatment is judged to have minimal benefits for a patient and may actually serve little purpose other than prolonging their existing poor health status, i.e. it is futile, then this gives added justification to allocating those resources to others for whom more positive outcomes are judged to be probable. Thus while cost should not be the main basis for decisions about which treatments to give, futility may provide a rationale for diverting resources.

In addition to, and closely linked to, the principle of justice, are two further principles subsidiary to the principle of respect for persons, which are of particular importance in health care. These are the principles of *beneficence* and *non-maleficence*, both of which have been alluded to in earlier chapters, and will be discussed more fully in the next chapter.

BENEFICENCE

According to Frankena (1963), the principle of beneficence can be summed up as follows:

> 1, One ought not to inflict evil or harm (what is bad); 2, One ought to prevent evil or harm; 3, One ought to remove evil; and 4, One ought to do or promise good. These four things are different, but they may appropriately be regarded as parts of the principle of beneficence.

In essence, the principle of beneficence is about doing good. The question then is, Would always *doing good* for the patient always result in justice? Not, the answer is, if in so doing one prohibits their autonomy. For, if patients have autonomy, then there could well be conflict between the idea that the professional should always do what is good for them, and what they want. What if what the patient wants is not what the professional judges to be good for them? Suppose it is decided that the best course of action – best, that is, in the interests of the patient's health – is that they should undergo surgery, but the patient, having been informed of the pros and cons of surgery, decides not to submit to it? Suppose they decide instead to discharge themselves? What, then, is the most just action? The question is: Is it more just to do what the patient wants, or what the health professional thinks is in their best interests?

If justice is to do with respect for persons, then to allow them personal autonomy is just. On the other hand, if justice (in health care) is about ensuring that individuals get what will be best for them, then it could be argued that to restrain them and give them the treatment would be just. The difficulty is in determining what is in the patient's best interests. It could be argued that what is in the best interests of any individual is allowing them autonomy, allowing them to decide for themselves which course of action to take. It might not be the 'healthiest' decision, but it might be the most just.

NON-MALEFICENCE

'Among the shibboleths of traditional medical ethics is the injunction "Primum non nocere" – first (or above all) do no harm' (Gillon, 1986). The question we ask here is, Would acting always in such a way as to do no harm to a patient be just? Obviously, in many instances this principle does accord with the principle of justice, if only because to do harm to someone is likely to do them an injustice. However, if to tell a patient the truth about their condition is considered harmful, then to fail to tell them would be in accordance with the principle of non-maleficence. Indeed, this is often the reason given for not telling patients their prognosis. However, as has already been claimed, to fail to tell or to withhold the truth from someone can be said to be treating them unjustly.

So it appears that while, on the face of it, the principles of beneficence and non-maleficence appear to uphold a notion of justice, both of them, if rigorously applied, can lead to injustice. The only real justice in our dealing with individuals is to treat them as autonomous moral beings, able and entitled to decide for themselves what is in their own best interests. It is also to treat them with respect, as equals with ourselves. One of the criticisms of the principles of beneficence and non-maleficence, as we shall see in the next chapter, is that they can lead to paternalism: the idea that one person knows what is best for another. This is clearly at odds with the above idea of justice.

SUMMARY

In this chapter we have explored the notion of justice as it pertains to health care. What clearly emerges is that justice, in the sense of fairness of distribution, is probably unattainable in health care. However, in view of the fact that absolute justice in health care may not be realistic, there is no moral justification for not striving to achieve it. Similarly, it would seem that in the one-to-one, professional–client situation, justice is something which is seldom achieved. Again, however, there is no moral justification for not trying to achieve it. In our dealings with individuals the most just action is to treat them with respect: to respect their value as another human being, and to afford to them moral respect. If in our dealings with others, be they patients or colleagues, we apply basic moral principles, such as truth-telling and promise-keeping, then that is to be just with them.

NOTE

1. RAWP reported in 1976, and its recommendations have greatly influenced allocation of resources to Regions ever since. Allocations are based on a formula which takes into account the age/sex distribution of the population weighted by the Standardized Mortality Ratio for the Region. In consequence, resources have over a period of time been transferred from those Regions deemed to be over-funded to those deemed to be under-funded.

REFERENCES

Downie, R.S. & Calman, K.C. (1987) *Healthy Respect – Ethics in Health Care.* London: Faber & Faber.

Frankena, W.K. (1963) cited in Seedhouse, D. (1988) *Ethics: the Heart of Health Care.* Chichester: J. Wiley & Sons.

Gillon, R. (1986) *Philosophical Medical Ethics.* Chichester: J. Wiley & Sons.

Seedhouse, D. (1988) *Ethics in Health Care.* Chichester: J. Wiley & Sons.

Spritz, N. (1997) Physicians and medical futility: experience in the setting of general medical care. In Zucker, M.B. & Zucker, H.D. (eds) *Medical Futility and the Evaluation of Life-sustaining Interventions.* Cambridge: Cambridge University Press.

Stockwell, F. (1972) *The Unpopular Patient.* London: RCN.

Townsend, P. *et al.* (1990) *Inequalities in Health Care and the Health Divide.* Harmondsworth: Penguin.

Williams, A. (1985) cited in Seedhouse, D. (1988) *Ethics in Health Care.* Chichester: J. Wiley & Sons.

FURTHER READING

Benjamin, M. & Curtis, J. (1992) *Ethics in Nursing,* 3rd edn. New York: Oxford University Press.

See Chapter 7 'Cost Containment, Justice and Rationing'.

14

Beneficence, non-maleficence and autonomy

In this chapter we return to three important ethical principles which have been touched on in previous chapters. These are the principles of *beneficence, non-maleficence* and *respect for autonomy*. What we will be concerned with in this chapter are three essential questions. First, what do the notions of beneficence and non-maleficence mean? Second, are they compatible or contradictory? And third, what is the relationship between both and the concept of patient autonomy?

BENEFICENCE

In the previous chapter I gave as a definition of beneficence that of Frankena. More simply, it is often seen as a moral injuction always to do good. In terms of health care that has tended to be interpreted in two ways, first the idea that one should always do what is best for the patient, and second, that the good of the patient should be put before one's own needs.

Let us now try to unpack these ideas. We will take them in reverse order, beginning with the idea of putting the patient's needs above our own.

'Among the more pious remarks to be heard in discussion of medical ethics is, "The patient's interests always come first"' (Gillon, 1986). Gillon is, of course talking about doctors, but the same notion holds true for nurses, midwives and other health workers. It is the thinking which lies behind the idea that nurses, unlike shop assistants, for example, do not go off duty on the bell if there is still work to be done. Obviously it would be difficult to justify leaving a patient when one is in the middle of carrying out some aspect of their care because it's the end of the shift. On the other hand, why should nurses feel obliged to stay on because either they, for very good reasons, have not finished their work or there is a shortage of staff on the next shift?

Now, it could be argued, though not very convincingly, that nurses have a duty to care, and that therefore they should remain on duty until they have carried out the care expected of them. On the other hand, it can be argued that the duty to care, in terms of giving care, only applies during the nurse's period of duty. The nurse's duty to care does extend beyond the period of duty, inasmuch as they have a responsibility to ensure that those to whom they hand over the care are fully informed of the patients' needs, what care has been given and the care they still require. It can also be argued that they have a responsibility to ensure the standards of continuing care by ascertaining that those to whom they hand over have adequate knowledge and skills. It would be difficult to justify a nurse going off duty if there was no one sufficiently qualified to whom the responsibility of caring for the patients could be passed. On the other hand, there is no moral obligation for the sort of extreme altruism, whereby nurses place the needs of patients above their own at all times, which we began by discussing, and which nurses are often made to feel they should practise.

The requirement to put the patient's interests first does not mean some extreme notion of self-sacrifice. It does mean, however, that some things may have to be sacrificed for it. Patients' needs can clearly be placed above organizational needs. Giving care to patients is of a higher priority than carrying out administrative tasks which have no direct effect on patient care, or attending meetings.

What, then, of the idea of always doing what is best for the patient?

Indeed, the extent to which beneficence or doing good for others is morally obligatory is vigorously debated by the theorists, and some even argue that there is no such moral obligation, though they usually hasten to add that beneficence is undoubtedly a virtue and morally commendable.

(Gillon, 1986)

Whether or not the principle is accepted in general ethics, it seems to me that in health care ethics it is more or less taken as read. It has its foundations in the Hippocratic Oath: 'I will follow that system or regimen which, according to my ability and judgement I consider for the benefit of my patients.' The idea is followed through in more modern codes, such as the *The Declaration of Geneva*, 1948, and reiterated in 1968 and 1983, and, of course, in the UKCC Code of Conduct (1992): 'Act always in such a way as to promote and safeguard the well-being and interests of patients/clients.'

That any nurse, or other health care professional, would want to act in any way other than for the benefit of the patient or client is not under debate. The crucial questions are: *Who decides what is in the patient's/client's best interests, and on what basis?* Two of the principal constraints against or criticisms of beneficence are that (1) it implies paternalism, and (2) it may conflict with the principle of justice.

BENEFICENT PATERNALISM

This term is often to be found in medical ethical writing. It is used generally in a positive and virtuous vein. Firstly, the doctor, because of his or her education and experience, *knows* what is best for the patient. And, since the doctor has a moral obligation to do good, then to determine on behalf of the patient what will be done to them is morally justified. In any case, there are those patients, such as the unconscious and the mentally handicapped, who are incapable of making informed decisions. However, it is important that the doctor or nurse in applying the duty of beneficence takes into account the wants and wishes of the patient. As we shall see later, the duty of beneficence must be tempered by the duty of respect for autonomy.

Secondly, the good of one patient cannot be seen in isolation. In doing good for one, we need to be sure that it is not to the detriment of others. The duty to do good is a duty to do good to all patients equally. The duty of beneficence needs to be tempered by the duty of justice. Herein, of course, lies a dilemma. How can a nurse do what is best for each and every individual? Is it always possible to do good for one person, without doing less than good for another? If patients have equal rights, is it possible for each to exert those rights to the full? In Chapter 6, it was noted that the freedom to exert one's rights may be restricted by the rights of others, that we can only exert our rights to the extent to which they do not impinge upon the rights of others. Thus, while within the individual nurse–patient relationship it is both appropriate and possible for a nurse to apply the principle of beneficence, when dealing with a group of patients, the nurse may have to decide what actions will result in the most good for all. To achieve this it may be necessary not to do all that any one individual might deserve or need. The question might be, not how to do good for a patient, but how to do the least harm to them.

NON-MALEFICENCE

'As a registered nurse, midwife or health visitor, you ... must: ensure that no action or omission on your part, or within your sphere of responsibility, is detrimental to the interests, condition or safety of patients and clients' (UKCC, 1992). This, the second clause in the Code of Conduct, arises out of the principle of non-maleficence, the idea that nurses have a duty not to harm patients or clients. But what exactly do we mean by that?

Many nursing activities, as medical ones, are in themselves harmful. To puncture a person's skin with a needle, or to insert a tube into one or other orifice, is to harm. At least, it certainly causes hurt and injury. Many procedures carry with them the risk of harm. Vaccinations and immunizations, for example, carry a risk, albeit in most cases a minimal risk, of causing harm. If the principle were to be taken to its extreme – *above all, do no harm* – then it would be difficult to justify the carrying out of a great number of medical and nursing procedures.

This raises the question: Why *above all?* Why should not doing harm be seen as taking priority over doing good? As Gillon (1986) points out, there is no sound historical evidence to support the claim at all. In fact, it is in no way certain from where the idea originated. That apart, can we morally defend the claim that the principle of not doing harm is the greater priority?

Consider the example, mentioned above, of giving vaccinations. We give vaccinations in order to do good. The intention is that vaccinations will benefit both the individual and the public. The benefit to the individual is that they will not contract the disease, and to the public that with every individual vaccinated the likelihood of the spread of the disease is diminished. However, there is a risk. A minority of people may suffer harmful side-effects – side-effects which can be very serious, even fatal.

If the prime duty is not to do harm, then, it could be argued that one should not give a vaccination to an individual, in order to prevent the possibility of harm to them. But, it could be counter-argued that in not giving the vaccination we also put them at risk of harm – that they contract the disease, the effects of which might be just as serious as the side-effects of the vaccination. Furthermore, we not only place that individual at risk, but also the wider community. Some would defend the decision not to give the vaccination on the grounds that inaction carries less moral weight than action.

To apply the principle 'above all, do no harm' in the case of giving vaccinations is clearly illogical. For it would mean not vaccinating anyone, and that would have obvious harmful effects. The case for doing something which carries a risk of harm, but is more likely to benefit not only the individual but the wider community, would appear to carry more weight.

Nevertheless, there are situations in which the injunction not to do harm will take precedence over the injunction to do good. A great many medical interventions carry with them risks. If the risks are high, and of a serious nature, then it can be argued that to carry out the treatment is morally indefensible. It comes back to applying the principle of double effect which we discussed in Chapter 2. In fact some (such as Foot, 1967), use the principle of double effect to substantiate the claim that not doing harm takes precedence over doing good, and she concludes: 'other things being equal, the obligation not to harm people is more stringent than the obligation to benefit people'.

It can also, as Gillon points out, be argued that to claim a duty not to do harm to anybody is more coherent than to claim a duty always to do good to everybody. The former is possible, while the latter is impossible. 'Thus at most we can have a duty to benefit some other people (an imperfect duty), while we have a perfect duty to everybody not to harm them' (Gillon, 1986). However, to argue from this that, when faced with a choice between doing good and not doing harm, not doing harm takes precedence is fallacious.

While there would seem to be no real reason for accepting the idea of *primum non nocere* (*first* do no harm) as holding any weight, there still remains the notion of a principle of not doing harm. It may not always take precedence, but it none the less is a principle to be applied. Just as with the principle of beneficence, there are constraints. The principle of not doing harm needs also to be tempered with the notion of patient autonomy and the principle of justice.

There is the same danger here, as with the principle of beneficence, that the doctor or nurse might be guilty of paternalism – that is, deciding on behalf of the patient or client what should not be done to them on the basis that it might or will harm them. Does not the patient or client have a right to decide for themselves whether or not to take the risk, or the extent of risk they are prepared to take? Also, as in the case of vaccination, there is the question of whether one is justified in taking a particular course of action to avoid doing harm to an individual at the risk of harming others.

BENEFICENCE AND NON-MALEFICENCE – THE RELATIONSHIP

As we have already seen, it is not possible to view these two principles separately. They are clearly intertwined. It can be argued that the principle of non-maleficence is not a principle in its own right, but merely an idea encompassed by the principle of beneficence. That is to say that not doing harm is an inevitable consequence of doing good. It would, after all, seem logical to claim that in doing good for someone, we cannot be doing them harm. But is this necessarily so?

As we have already noted, in many medical and nursing interventions aimed at doing good, there is an element of doing harm. Sometimes, the harm is unavoidable, even intentional – as in the case of surgery. At other times it is unintended and unexpected (unexpected, that is, inasmuch as it is an undocumented or extremely rare side-effect). In between these two positions, there is the unintended, but known, possibility of a harmful side-effect. To help clarify the arguments, let us consider an example falling within each of these three.

First, to amputate someone's leg is to do them harm. However, if the reason for so doing is that they are suffering from gangrene, then to do so is beneficent, for it will prevent further harm, and in some situations might be life-saving. In such a case, as in so many medical and nursing situations, to do harm in order to benefit the patient is justifiable.

To tell the truth is an accepted moral principle. Normally, telling a patient the truth about their diagnosis and prognosis is not expected to have major harmful effects. It might make them depressed or anxious. It might make them 'give up'. But all these effects might be expected, though not intended or desired, and can be overcome with skilled counselling. There might be an unexpected outcome. The patient might have a heart attack and die. Such an event would obviously be unintentional, and also be unexpected. Patients do not usually react in this way even when the information is of a very disturbing nature. Such an occurrence would not be a reason for arguing that it was wrong to tell the truth.

So, what of the middle position – the one over which there is perhaps more cause for debate? The majority of medical, and a considerable number of nursing, treatments carry a degree of risk. All drugs have known side-effects. In some the side-effects are rare but serious; in others they are very common but not very serious. Giving an enema can have harmful side-effects – there is a risk of damage to tissue, and that the patient might go into a state of shock. Catheterization can also cause tissue damage, and there is always the risk of introducing infection, and, less common, the risk of perforating the urethra. Are we then to argue, on the grounds of first do no harm, that treatments which carry known risks should not be given?

Suppose that 90% of patients who are catheterized contract a urinary tract infection. Could we justify ever catheterizing anyone? Certainly, it would be difficult to justify catheterizing people as a way of managing incontinence. The principle of non-maleficence would hold, since we would be replacing one distressing complaint with another equally distressing one. On the other hand, if a patient has urinary retention, then the duty to do good would dictate that the patient be catheterized. In this case the harmful effects of not acting outweigh those of acting.

Thus, we begin to see that in some instances doing good and not doing harm amount to more or less the same thing, while in others one has to make a choice between doing good and not doing harm. In some of these situations doing good might actually cause harm, but the good is considered to outweigh the harm. And in some instances, where the harm outweighs the good, then the duty not to harm takes precedence over the duty to do good. In the end, the morally justified act is that which causes the least harm and the most good.

AUTONOMY

In the foregoing discussion we were concerned with how the nurse or doctor might decide on the best course of action. There was, deliberately, no mention of the patient, other than as the subject of the action. However, as was noted earlier, the principles of beneficence and non-maleficence must be tempered by respect for autonomy. What, though, do we mean by autonomy? And in particular what do we mean by the autonomy of the patient?

Autonomy can be defined as 'the capacity to think, decide, and act on the basis of such thought and decision freely and independently and without let or hindrance' (Gillon, 1986). Autonomy does not mean freedom to do as one wants or to act in accordance with one's desires. Autonomous action is based on rational thought or reason. It embodies the notions of freedom and liberty, but only within the constraints of reason.

Respect for autonomy

Most, if not all, of us would accept the idea that we should respect the autonomy of others, if for no other reason than we would want them to respect ours. However, we might not want that respect to be absolute. Both these views find support in the major schools of ethical thought. Kant, for example, argues that respect for autonomy is a universal law, and is supported both by the *categorical imperative* (see Ch. 2, Note 2), and the concept of respect for persons. However, he argued that respect for the autonomy of any one individual had to be seen within the context of respect for the autonomy of all. Similarly, utilitarians, such as Mill, also support the principle of respect for autonomy. The utilitarian argument is that such respect would maximize human happiness. If individuals are allowed the freedom to act autonomously they will be happier, and the sum total of happiness will be increased. However, the utilitarians too do not see it as being absolute. They argue that the obligation to respect people's autonomy holds only as long as it does not cause harm to others.

The autonomy of the patient

We turn now to the application of the general concept of autonomy and the principle of respect for autonomy to the health care situation, and, in particular, to the relationship between the principles of beneficence and non-maleficence and the principle of respect for autonomy.

In Chapter 9, it was suggested that the nurse has a role to play in maintaining the patient's autonomy. Now, given that autonomy is the ability to decide an act on the basis of reason, it follows that if the patient is to be able to exert any autonomy, then they must be given the necessary information in order to do so. If their autonomy is to be respected, then health professionals have to allow patients to make decisions and act upon them.

Herein lie two possible areas of conflict. Firstly, since it is the health professional who has the information, they can determine the amount of information the patient will receive. Secondly, the patient may decide to act in a way which the health professional considers not to be in their best interests. Gorovitz *et al.* (1976) write: 'acts of interference with other persons' autonomy are often justified by the claim that the acts are for the benefit or welfare of those who are being interfered with'. The principle of beneficence is seen as taking precedence over the principle of respect for autonomy.

Often, health professionals will claim to be allowing patients to make informed decisions about their treatment and care while only providing them with that information which means they will almost certainly elect the choice of action which the professional considers to be the best one. The choice offered is between the treatment the professionals consider best and no treatment. The patient is thus presented with a choice between possible cure, and no cure. Or, when alternatives are put forward there is a strong bias in favour of the professionals' preference. The professional would defend such action on the basis that they were acting in the patient's best interests, and preventing harm. That is fair enough, provided they acknowledge what they are doing, which is restricting the patient's autonomy. If the professional claims that they are respecting the patient's autonomy by giving them choice, then they delude themselves and deceive the patient.

In the previous paragraph, I have deliberately referred to the health professional, because there is an erroneous tendency to think that it is only doctors who are guilty of such coercive paternalism. Nurses, midwives and other health care workers can be equally guilty. Sometimes, their guilt lies in supporting the doctor's decisions and actions, but at other times the decisions are theirs. For example, a health visitor might claim to be allowing the client autonomous choice when discussing vaccination. However, if what the health visitor does is to explain the probable benefits of the vaccine, and possible harmful consequences of not having the vaccine, then he or she has not told the whole story.

On other occasions, nurses will employ other tactics which, although intended only to benefit and not harm the patient, do reduce their autonomy. 'Patients are expected to turn, cough, breathe deeply, get out of bed, and urinate, for example, on the nurse's command' (Bandman and Bandman, 1990). Such commands, especially when accompanied by some form of threat: 'If you don't get out of bed now, you'll have to wait until lunchtime, because I will be too busy before then', are an affront to the patient's autonomy because they reduce the degree of voluntariness on the part of the patient. An autonomous action is one which is undertaken voluntarily, and not under coercion, however covert that coercion may be.

The real difficulty arises when the patient, having been given all the information, makes a choice which the health professional considers not to be in their best interest. This can pose a very real dilemma for nurses and midwives. For the Code of Conduct states that they shall 'Act always in such a way as to promote and safeguard the well-being and interests of patient/clients', while at the same time 'Take account of the customs, values and spiritual beliefs of patients/clients'.

There are two issues here. Firstly, what is in the patient's/client's best interests? That they undergo the treatment or care which the nurse, midwife or health visitor considers to be in their best interests, or that their autonomy be respected? Secondly, there may well be conflict between acting in their best interests, and respecting their customs, values and spiritual beliefs.

There is no all-embracing answer to either of these conflicts. Each situation has to be judged on its own merits. In some situations it would be right for the principle of beneficence to override respect for autonomy, and in others vice versa. Similarly, it might be more appropriate to act in the patient's best interests even if this means going against their customs, values or beliefs; while in other situations it might be more appropriate to respect those customs, values or beliefs even if the result may not be in what we consider their best interests.

Suppose, for example, an in-patient, who is suffering from chronic emphysema, having been fully informed of all the consequences, decides that they will carry on smoking? That is their autonomous decision. Do we respect it? Or would we be justified in preventing them from obtaining cigarettes? It could be argued that the most beneficent action would be to prevent them from obtaining cigarettes, or at least ensuring that they never had opportunity to smoke by confining them to a non-smoking area. This would to some extent alleviate their symptoms and slow up the progress of their disease. On the other hand, since their life is going to be pretty miserable whether they smoke or not (and smoking might actually provide them with some pleasure), then, for them to choose to act in a way which might increase their problems and shorten their life is their right. We might think it foolish, but they have a right to make that decision. However, the exercise of autonomy assumes a degree of rationality. And, it could be argued that, having been given all the available information, to decide to continue to smoke is irrational, and therefore not a true exercise of moral autonomy at all. Thus, it could be concluded that the nurses would be justified in this case to give precedence to the principle of beneficence.

What, though, if the 'best' treatment contradicts the patient's religious values or beliefs? Consider, for example, the case of a Jehovah's Witness who refuses a blood transfusion, which is considered necessary as an integral part of their treatment. I am talking here of an adult, not a child. (This issue in relation to the children of Jehovah's Witnesses has been much written about, and we shall touch on it in the next chapter.) Here we are concerned with an adult, in full possession of all their faculties who, although consenting to all other aspects of their prescribed treatment, refuses to have a blood transfusion on religious grounds.

Recourse to the principle of non-maleficence would suggest that the patient's desires be overridden, since to give the blood transfusion would prevent harm occurring to the patient. This would clearly contravene the principle of respect for autonomy. The principle of beneficence, on the one hand, could be evoked to justify giving the blood transfusion despite the patient's wishes, since to do so would be to promote their health. Any action which promotes health must be beneficent. On the other hand, the principle of beneficence could be used to justify not giving the transfusion, on the grounds that this would be respecting the patient's right to choose. And respecting a person's right to choose is to respect their autonomy and so to respect them as a person. Allowing a person to maintain their autonomy, it could be argued, is a beneficent act.

In this, as in most moral dilemmas, there is no clear cut answer. The individual has to decide for him- or herself which is the overriding principle. If respect for autonomy is seen as being the overriding principle and the patient, despite advice to the contrary, insists on refusing the transfusion, then we have to abide by that choice. However, the surgeon would be quite justified in then refusing to carry out the operation, if in his or her opinion to do so without giving a blood transfusion would put the patient's life at risk – that is, if the consequences of operating without transfusing are likely to be more harmful than the consequences of not operating.

SUMMARY

In this chapter we have been concerned with three moral principles of particular relevance to health care ethics: *beneficence, non-maleficence* and *respect for autonomy*. Beneficence, the principle of only acting for the good of the patient, and non-maleficence, the principle of not doing harm, are likely in most situations to be in accord. However, as we have seen, there are situations in which conflict can arise. Since both principles can lead to a paternalistic approach, they are frequently in conflict with the principle of respect for autonomy.

It can, however, be argued that to respect a person's autonomy is in itself beneficent. For, as was argued in Chapter 1, to deny someone their autonomy is to treat them as less than a whole person, it is in effect a non-beneficent act. If autonomy is seen as an integral element of health or wholeness, then to respect autonomy is to allow a person one of the attributes which is part of functioning as a whole person. It is to enable them to achieve health or wholeness. If, as Seedhouse (1988) argues, health is in itself morally good, then any action which enhances health must be morally good. Respecting autonomy is thus a beneficent act in itself because it is a necessary element in achieving the overall goal – health.

Issues for discussion

Mr B, aged 72, was admitted to hospital two weeks ago having been found by a neighbour lying on his kitchen floor in a 'drowsy and confused' state. On admission he was found to be suffering from a chest infection and anaemia. Both these conditions have now been resolved, but throughout his hospital stay Mr B has remained mildly confused and forgetful. He has frequently been unable to find his own bed, and forgotten to do simple tasks. The consultant considers that Mr B is not capable of caring for himself and should be discharged not to his own home but to a nursing home.

The occupational therapist (OT) has carried out a home assessment with Mr B and considers that with support from a home carer he would be able to manage safely in his own home. The OT suggests a variety of simple safety measures such as a clear notice by the gas cooker to remind him to turn off the gas.

The consultant remains unconvinced and still insists in the interests of Mr B's safety that he be discharged to a nursing home. Mr B, however, is extremely reluctant to comply with this and insists that he be allowed to return to his own home. He says that having visited his home with the OT he is aware of the possible dangers and knows how to avoid these.

Which course of action would be most beneficent? Should Mr B be transferred to a nursing home for his own safety, or should his autonomy be respected and, despite the possible risks of harm to himself, he be allowed to return to his own home?

REFERENCES

Bandman, E.L. & Bandman, B. (1990) *Nursing Ethics through the Life Span,* 2nd edn. Englewood Cliffs: Prentice-Hall.

Foot, P. (1967) The problem of abortion and the principle of double effect. *Oxford Review,* 5, 5–15.

Frankena, W.K. (1963) cited in Seedhouse, D. (1988) *Ethics; the Heart of Health Care.* Chichester: J. Wiley & Sons.

Gillon, R. (1986) *Philosophical Medical Ethics.* Chichester: J. Wiley & Sons.

Gorovitz, S. *et al.* (1976) *Moral Problems in Medicine.* Englewood Cliffs, NJ: Prentice-Hall.

Kant, I. *Critique of Pure Reason.* In Kemp Smith, N. (ed.) (1973) *Immanuel Kant's Critique of pure Reason.* London: Macmillan.

Seedhouse, D. (1988) *Ethics: the Heart of Health Care.* Chichester: J. Wiley & Sons.

UKCC (United Kingdom Central Council for Nursing, Midwifery and Health Visiting) (1992) *Code of Professional Conduct for the Nurse, Midwife and Health Visitor,* 3rd edn. London: UKCC.

World Medical Association (1983) *Declaration of Geneva.* Geneva: WMA.

FURTHER READING

In addition to the above references, see also:

An End to the Benevolent Conspiracy: Nurses' and Patients' Rights. Hastings Centre Report 11 (October 1981): 3–4.

Beauchamp, T.L. & Childress, J.P. (1983) *Principles of Biomedical Ethics,* 2nd edn. Oxford: Oxford University Press.

15

The vulnerable patient

It may appear strange that this chapter should be entitled 'the vulnerable patient' when, as was previously suggested in Chapters 6 and 9, patients are vulnerable by virtue of the fact that they are patients. However, some groups of patients may be more vulnerable than others, because of their age, condition/disease or gender. In this chapter we shall be concerned with some of those groups of patients who are more vulnerable than others, and we shall discuss specific ethical issues in relation to each.

The groups and issues we shall discuss are these: children and informed consent; persons with learning disabilities and autonomy; female patients and paternalism; and sufferers of AIDS and respect for persons.

CHILDREN AND INFORMED CONSENT

It is custom and practice in the United Kingdom to obtain the consent of a parent or guardian to carry out treatment on a minor. I deliberately use the phrase 'custom and practice' because there is no reason in law in England and Wales[1] why a minor may not give consent to treatment, and there are strong moral arguments why they should.

Perhaps first we need to decide what is meant by a child. The answer to this is not as simple as it might seem. As Wieczorek and Natopoff (1981) point out, the length, essential nature and meaning of childhood are culturally determined. Thus in one society a child may be defined in law as a person aged 12 years or under, while in another the upper age may be 16 years. The age of consent (to sexual intercourse), for example, varies from society to society. Similarly, the status of children within the family and society is subject to a variety of views. Bandman and Bandman (1990) suggest three models of parent–child relations.

The first is the *ownership* model in which children are perceived as being possessions of their parents. This is to deny the child any moral autonomy and to view them as having only a limited range of rights. While the ownership model might encompass notions of caring, nurturing and protection, it does limit the extent to which a child is enabled to develop his or her own set of values. In many ways this is the model applied in health care in the United Kingdom. It is the parents who are afforded the right to make decisions about treatment on behalf of their child, who may not be involved at all in the process. On the other hand, it does mean that when parents are seen to be failing in their duties towards the child, as in cases of neglect or abuse, the professionals can take over 'ownership' of the child for beneficent reasons.

The second model is the *partnership* model. Within this model the parent–child relationship is viewed as one of almost equality. Parents and child negotiate and agree actions. While the parents may still retain ultimate control, this model does permit the child to develop moral values and the ability to reason. The application of this model to health care would suggest that the relationship between nurse, child and parents should also be seen as one of a partnership. It affords to the child the same rights as those of any other patient – to be fully involved in the decision-making process about their care. This model, it will be argued, is the most morally acceptable one for the nurse to adopt.

The third model is that of *club membership*. In this model all members of the family, although owing some responsibility to the maintenance of the family, are not cared for very much as individuals. Each family member, adult or child, is left very much to their own devices and there is likely to be little parental guidance. The child, while given the freedom to make their own choices, is not always provided with the necessary guidelines or moral framework to make decisions.

The partnership model would appear to be the preferable one in that it combines the caring, nurturing and protective attributes of the ownership model with the freedom to develop as an individual of the club membership model. At the same time it repudiates some of the less acceptable attributes of the other two models. In effect, it treats the child as an individual and as a morally autonomous person who is encouraged and enabled to make their own choices and decisions.

The next questions are these: What are the necessary attributes to make decisions, such as consenting to or refusing treatment, and at what age do children become capable of so doing? In order to make such decisions three attributes are required:

1. Possession of a set of values and goals
2. The ability to communicate and understand information
3. The ability to reason and deliberate about one's choice.

(The President's Commission, 1982)

While one might debate the extent to which some adults possess all these attributes, what concerns us here is the age at which they are normally acquired. Certainly, there is no evidence to support the idea that they do not exist below the age of 16 years, nor are they suddenly evident at that age. Moral development, as all other aspects of development (physical, mental, social and emotional), varies from one individual to another.

Thus, it may well be that some children at a considerably earlier age than 16 years may have developed, at least to a reasonable degree, the three attributes mentioned above. Clearly, the infant will not possess any of them, but some children from the age of 7 years (the age traditionally known as 'the age of reason' – the age at which a child is able to differentiate between right and wrong) may well have developed these attributes to a sufficient degree at least to be able to participate in the decision-making process.

If we are to consider children as persons like any others, rather than as almost a separate species, then we have to allow them to make a contribution to discussions about their care. The partnership model described above facilitates this. In this model the child becomes a partner with his or her parents and the nurse in deciding whether to consent to or refuse treatment. To apply the ownership model is to deny that the child is a person in their own right, and to apply the club membership model is to be irresponsible. 'The partnership model of relationship recognises children as full human beings due respect for their thoughts, feelings, interests, and desires in relation to their own health care' (Bandman and Bandman, 1990).

Bandman and Bandman (1990) go on to say, 'Ideally, the

Partnership Model of relationships is based on an open, shared decision-making process, in which children's growing autonomy is supported to the extent of each child's cognitive maturation, personality, and thought processes.' The nurse then first needs, as part of her assessment of the child as a patient, to assess the extent to which they have developed a set of values and goals and to which they are capable of communicating and understanding information and thinking about the consequences of particular choices of action. Having – though it is far from easy – assessed the stage of the child's moral development, the nurse can then involve the child as fully as possible in the decision-making process. This means communicating information about his or her condition and its treatment in terms that the child can fully understand. Furthermore, it may also mean that when necessary – for example, when there is evidence of strong parental control and interference – the nurse may need to invoke the role as patient advocate, giving support to the child and enabling the child to express their own feelings. For there will be situations in which the parents' ideas may not be in the child's best interests, and the paramount role of the nurse, as has been noted in earlier chapters, is to act always in the interests of the patient.

There will be cases in which the child's wishes should be overruled: for example, a child who has taken an overdose of medication, or has swallowed some poisonous substance. In such a case, even though the child refuses to consent, the nurse would be justified in agreeing with the parent's wishes that appropriate treatment be carried out. On other occasions it would be morally defensible to either ignore the parent's wishes or not even seek their consent. If a girl of 14, for example, having contracted venereal disease, seeks treatment and does not wish her parents to know, then she has every right to consent to that treatment and have her privacy respected. Other situations are perhaps less clear. What, for example, of the 12-year-old suffering from carcinoma who does not want to undergo the amputation of a limb, the intention of which is to prolong life? Should the nurse support the child's wishes or those of the parents that the operation be carried out?

If we are to treat children, assuming they demonstrate the three attributes noted earlier, in the same way as we would an adult in such a situation, should we not afford them the same rights?

Bandman and Bandman (1990) contend that in such a situation the parent, 'invoking the principle of preventing greater harm, has the right to override the child's right to refuse'. However, there is a danger in pursuing this idea, for it would, if taken to its logical conclusion, mean that no patient has the ultimate right to refuse treatment. For, if the patient were an adult rather than a child, it could be argued that the doctor has the same right to override the patient's wishes on the basis of the same moral principle.

The question of the age at which a person should be able to consent freely to or refuse treatment is further compounded in the United Kingdom by the anomalous position of 16- and 17-year-olds. 16- and 17-year-olds fall between two stools: in the eyes of the law they are not children nor are they adults. This point was illustrated in 1992 when the Appeal Court ruled that in the case of a 16-year-old girl suffering from anorexia nervosa a doctor had the right to force-feed her against her wishes. The argument was that, as a result of her condition, she was not capable of making a rational decision. Now this may be so, but it might equally be a case of deciding the patient's ability to make that choice after they have made it (see Ch. 9). The girl may have made that decision at an earlier stage when it might have been assessed that she was capable of making a rational decision. Furthermore, had she consented to the treatment, then her ability to make such a decision would not have been called into question. The implications of the Court's decision are far-reaching, for what it might be doing is extending the notional age at which a person may consent to or refuse treatment to 18 years.

In this section we have been concerned with the principle of informed consent as it applies to children. Little has been said about the principle itself, since that was discussed in Chapter 9; rather, discussion has centred on whether children are able to and should be allowed to consent to or refuse treatment. Essentially, the argument that has been put forward is that children are persons, and if capable of making reasoned decisions, have the right to be involved in the decision-making process. To do so means that they need to be fully informed in the same way as was argued earlier as all patients. It was also argued that a partnership model involving the nurse, parents and child as equal partners is the most appropriate one to adopt.

AUTONOMY AND PERSONS WITH LEARNING DISABILITIES

Before we can begin this discussion we need to define what is meant by autonomy and to distinguish between *autonomous persons* and *respecting autonomy*. Autonomy has been defined as 'the power of self-determination and freedom from alien domination and constraint' (Smith, 1967). It is, then, about independence and freedom to choose, and about not being coerced into doing something one would not otherwise choose to do. Now, clearly, some persons cannot exercise autonomy. Young infants and the comatose are not able to either make or express choices.

Some would argue that for someone to be defined as an autonomous person they must possess certain attributes. These include *possession of consciousness, a self-concept, self-awareness, the capacity to reason, to be able to plan ahead, to be able to choose freely and the ability to direct his own life* (Feinberg, 1982; Seedhouse, 1988). Thus, if possession of all, or even most of these attributes is essential to the definition of an autonomous person, then it could be claimed that a large number of people with severe learning disabilities do not qualify. That is why we need to make the distinction between being an autonomous person and respecting autonomy. For to respect a person's autonomy is to allow them, within their capabilities, the freedom to choose for themselves.

Because, according to Seedhouse (1988), the aim of health care is to help the patient become independent, therefore the creation of autonomy is essential to the practice of all health work: 'health intervention is done in order to allow the person the widest possible degree of autonomy'. Thus, in the case of people with learning disabilities who might be judged by the criteria identified above as not being autonomous, the role of the health worker is to enable them to acquire a greater degree of autonomy. It means helping them develop skills to make choices and providing them with information in terminology which they can understand.

Creating autonomy, although central to health care, is not the same as respecting autonomy, although the one does relate to the other. For if we accept the idea that the creation of autonomy is central to health work, then having created it we must respect it.

> *The requirement to respect autonomy is a major part of the core rationale of health work, and it is significantly different from the necessity to create autonomy. The creation of autonomy requires the provision of the physical and mental wherewithal for rational self-direction, whereas respecting autonomy requires that the person's chosen direction should be respected, whether or not the health worker approves of that direction.*

(Seedhouse, 1988)

It is perhaps worth remembering that even persons whom we might judge as being capable of rational thought do make irrational decisions. We may try to change their minds, but at the end of the day we have to respect their decision. So too should we with those whom we might judge as having a lesser capability.

Persons with learning disabilities merit our respect as much as those whom we call 'normal'. We owe it to them to allow them that degree of feedom which is neither seriously harmful to themselves or to others. Yet frequently they are deprived of even some of the basic human freedoms. Society, through the courts, condones the compulsory sterilization of a 17-year-old girl with severe learning disabilities. The arguments are that she is incapable of making an informed decision, that were she to become pregnant she might not be able to comprehend what was happening to her, and that she would not be capable of providing for and caring for the child. Yet, an unmarried mother of five, who is socially deprived and perhaps of low intelligence, may be advised to undergo sterilization but is allowed to make her own choice. Is there actually that much difference between the two cases? In both cases the prospective mother may be incapable of adequately caring for her child and the burden of care may fall upon the State. The first may actually give more love to the child than the second, who may not really want the child and also be already under so much stress that she cannot provide the love that the child deserves. Yet in the one case we respect the woman's autonomy and in the other we do not. There is, in effect, very little rationality in the decisions we are making as a society.

It is not only about such dramatic issues as this that we disallow people with learning disabilities freedom to choose. Perhaps more than any other group they are denied, particularly in institutional care, the opportunity to make choices about very basic needs. The role of the nurse must be, firstly, to provide them with the information and freedom to make choices in activities of living, and, secondly, to act as advocate on their behalf in order that their choices be respected.

PATERNALISM AND WOMEN'S HEALTH

Passing reference has been made in previous chapters to the notion of paternalism. Here we explore that notion in greater detail and relate it to women's health, for nowhere in health care has paternalism been more assiduously applied than in the care of women. First, though, we begin by defining paternalism. The word *paternalism* is derived from the Latin – *pater*, meaning father – and literally means that *father knows best*. In health care ethics this is interpreted, as was noted in Chapter 5, as 'the doctor knows best' – in other words, that doctors, because of their superior knowledge, know better than the patient what is best for them. However, more importantly in the context under discussion here, it is that men know better than women.

Space does not permit a full discussion of the historical relationship between men and women in our culture. However, it is important to note that the medical profession has been and, despite the fairly recent entry into the profession of women, remains male-dominated. Since doctors define what is ill health – namely, what departs from the norm and requires their intervention – then because women are different from men biologically, medicine has defined what is normal for women as being abnormal.

> *Doctors developed the theory that woman's normal state was to be sick, because female functions were inherently pathological. This particularly applied to her monthly periods, which were seen as a sickness which necessitated rest and suspension of any physical activity such as long walks, dancing, riding and socialising.*

(Webb, 1987)

In the same way both pregnancy and the menopause were defined as 'ill health', whereas they are in reality part of normal, healthy processes. Women therefore became seen as being victims of their own bodies and needing help from doctors, who happened to be men. And, because they were unable to control these stages in their life cycle they needed men – who were normal and therefore superior – to 'treat' them.

Sadly, this attitude of male doctors towards female patients is still pervasive today, and 'women continue to be defined as appendages of their genital organs, with personalities which are inherently less active, ambitious, rational and intellectual than those of men (Webb, 1987).

To summarize, firstly, doctors define what constitutes ill health, which they have described as departure from the norm; secondly, that (since doctors are traditionally male) the 'norm' is all that which constitutes maleness and consequently being female is in itself abnormal; thirdly, that women are therefore sick by virtue of the fact that they are not male; and, perhaps most crucially here, fourthly, that because women are victims of their own bodies, they cannot help being 'sick'.

The final statement is crucial because it leads to the patting-on-the-head approach – 'Never mind, you can't help it, but I can help you'. This is frequently followed by 'Just take these pills'. This is, perhaps, an overstatement of reality, and will be questioned by doctors and patients alike. However, there is more than sufficient evidence to show that male doctors treat female patients in a very different way from that in which they treat male patients (Clarke, 1983; Smith, 1975). That being said, it should also be noted that doctors are not the only ones guilty of seeing women as being inferior. Male doctors are simply reflecting the attitudes of males generally towards females:

there is no psychology, no sociology, no anthropology of women. The problems and priorities of women are regarded as unimportant and main areas of women's lives such as childbirth and sexuality have only been examined if they pose problems for the male world.

(Orr, 1987)

What, then, is the role of the nurse in all this? This chapter is entitled 'The vulnerable patient'. This is not to suggest that women are more vulnerable than men because they are women, but what is being argued is that women, when they enter into the health-care system, become more vulnerable because of the way in which they are perceived by the male-dominated medical profession. The nurse's role then must be to ensure that a female patient (whatever her need for health care) receives the same response and care as a male patient. In this nurses are both advantaged and disadvantaged by the fact that nursing is predominantly a female profession. The advantage is that nurses are more likely to empathize with female patients, and are therefore able to question the conventional medical view of women and illness. The disadvantage is that nursing itself suffers from the historical relationship between men and women in society, and therefore may experience the same difficulties as women patients in disputing the views held by the medical profession.

The role of the nurse would seem to be two-fold: 'The feminist perspective demonstrates the needs for nurses to form stronger links with providers, and women as users of health care' (O'Connor, 1987). The nurse, then, firstly has a role in relation to women clients, be they carers or patients. The nurse's role is one of advocacy and empowerment. The nurse has a responsibility to promote the needs of women and to speak out against the way in which they are perceived and treated by the health-care system. The nurse should also be involved in helping women understand what is happening to them when they come into contact with the health-care system and in helping them develop the knowledge and skills to enable them to bring about change. The nurse has a role to play too in relation to other health-care workers, not least doctors, in educating them about the health-care needs of women. To fail to take on these roles is to fail to ensure that members of a particular client group receive considerate and appropriate care. All patients, regardless of gender, race or age, are entitled to expect to be treated as individual persons, and to receive care which is based on assessment of their needs as an individual rather than as a stereotypical member of a group.

RESPECT FOR PERSONS
– SUFFERERS FROM AIDS

In many ways all the themes we have so far explored in this chapter are encompassed by the principle of *respect for persons*. In Chapter 4 this notion was defined as meaning 'that any person, as such, has intrinsic worth or value irrespective of his achievements, which in the dealing of other persons with him, may be neither ignored or discounted' (Harris, 1966). I would want to expand this definition to say that not only is a person of worth or value irrespective of their achievements but also irrespective of their lack of achievements or lifestyle, and that therefore in our dealings with patients we should treat them all equally as having intrinsic worth and value.

The care of patients who have contracted human immunodeficiency virus (HIV) and/or are suffering from acquired immune deficiency syndrome (AIDS) poses several ethical issues. For the most part these arise out of two characteristics of the disease. Firstly, it is an infectious disease with no known cure. Secondly its acquisition is associated with particular lifestyles.

The emergence of HIV and AIDS has meant that the nursing and medical professions find themselves confronting a situation which was common to our predecessors some 50 or 100 years ago. Then nurses and doctors spent a great deal of their time in caring for patients who were suffering from highly contagious diseases for which there was no known cure. Since the advent of vaccines, antibiotics and other health-care innovations, it is not a situation which many practitioners have had to face. Nor is it something which Western society has had to face for several decades. Hence the notion of 'the 20th-century plague', and calls for isolation hospitals and even compulsory hospitalization of sufferers. Given this scenario, it is essential that the nurse does not allow patients to feel that they are being ostracized or treated as 'unclean'. The nurse also has a role to play in educating relatives and friends of the patient and the public at large particularly about the way in which the virus is communicated. There still remain a number of myths which need to be exploded.

A second consequence of the nature of the disease is that there is tremendous pressure to find a cure. The pressure comes from both the patients themselves and from society as a whole. What this inevitably gives rise to is the development of new drugs and the need to test them. Sufferers of AIDS are extremely vulnerable to suggestions that they try out new drugs, and may be so desperate for something which will ease their suffering and/or cure their disease that they will not question or listen to information about their treatment. The nurse has a vital role to play here in ensuring that consent is informed and freely given, and in counselling the patient both during and following the decision-making process.

Other issues arise out of the fact that the disease is associated, rightly or wrongly, with particular lifestyles. I intend here to highlight three issues. Firstly, there is the danger that the assumption will be made that every patient with the disease falls into one of the 'at-risk' categories, and assumptions made about him or her which are unfounded. The second issue is that because the disease is associated with particular lifestyles there is a danger of victim-blaming. The third issue is that when the patient does fall into one of the 'at-risk' groups they might be treated differently from other patients.

Firstly, then, we cannot assume that because a patient has contracted the virus that they may fall into one of the 'at-risk' groups. There is increasing evidence that many people may contract the virus who are neither homosexuals, promiscuous nor intravenous drug abusers. If they do not fall into one of these groups then they may be experiencing a range of feelings, not least anger towards the person from whom they contracted the disease, or, in the case of having been given a transfusion of infected blood, against the health service. The nurse must (1) ensure that patients are not inappropriately labelled; (2) offer a sympathetic ear to the patient, and (3) counsel the patient against giving vent to their anger against those whom they hold responsible for their condition.

In the case of those patients who do fall into one of the 'at-risk' groups there is always the risk that they may be made to feel guilty. While in a sense they do carry some degree of responsibility inasmuch as had they not adopted a particular lifestyle they might not have contracted the disease, they cannot be held entirely to blame – in just the same way as those who smoke, drink alcohol, take inadequate exercise or eat an inadequate diet cannot be entirely held to blame for the fact that they suffer from lung cancer, coronary heart disease or any other conditions associated with those types of behaviour. For while their behaviour or lifestyle may be a major contributory factor to their contracting the disease, the fact that they have behaved in that way may not be entirely of their own volition. There are a number of social, economic and political reasons which cause people to adopt an 'unhealthy' lifestyle. The individual cannot be held entirely to blame for their behaviour or its consequences. Nurses must guard against giving the impression to the patient that they hold them responsible for their illness, do all they can to ensure that others do not display a similar attitude and, perhaps most importantly, help the patient to overcome their feelings of guilt.

One of the questions I am frequently asked by groups of nurses is whether a nurse might make conscientious objection to nursing patients with AIDS. The answer is a definite 'No'. Conscientious objection may only be made to carrying out specific procedures which are either contrary to the nurse's moral beliefs and values or which the nurse feels are unnecessary and harmful to the patient. A nurse cannot, as has already been noted, refuse to care for a patient who has had an abortion; he or she may only decline to participate in the procedure.

But why should this question be asked? It may be that some nurses feel that there is a risk to themselves in caring for AIDS sufferers. However, the risk is only there if they do not follow safe procedures, and is in any case less than the risk of hepatitis B. The other reason is probably related to views about the 'type' of person who is likely to have contracted the disease. This is to make a moral judgement about a person, and to imply that some people are less worthy than others. A nurse cannot refuse to nurse a patient, be they homosexual, promiscuous, a prostitute or intravenous drug abuser simply because the nurse disapproves of their lifestyle. To do so is to impose his or her own moral values on patients, and to judge some as being of less worth than others. It is to lack respect for them as persons.

SUMMARY

In this chapter we have been concerned with four issues or themes – informed consent, autonomy, paternalism and respect for persons. As will have become apparent, these four issues are interrelated and could all be encompassed in the fourth – namely, respect for persons. For what we have been concerned with throughout this chapter is the moral imperative of treating each individual as a person in their own right.

While discussion of each issue has been related to a particular group of patients, it should also have become apparent that the principles discussed can and should be applied to all patients. The four groups of patients discussed were chosen because they are, at least within our health-care system, perhaps more vulnerable than other groups. This is not to say that they are the only vulnerable groups, and we could equally have considered others, such as elderly and mentally ill persons.

NOTE

1. In Scotland a child under the age of 16 years is not allowed to consent to treatment by law.
   See also discussion of the case of *Gillick* v *W. Norfolk and Wisbech Area Health Authority* (1986) in Tingle, J. and Cribb, A. (eds) (1995) *Nursing Law and Ethics*, pp. 200, 241–243.

REFERENCES

Bandman, E.L. & Bandman, B. (1990) *Nursing Ethics through the Life Span*. Englewood Cliffs, NJ: Prentice-Hall.

Clarke, J.M. (1983) Sexism, feminism and medicalism: a decade review of literature on gender and illness. *Sociology of Health and Illness*, 5(1), 62–82.

Feinberg, J. (1982) The problem of personhood. In Beauchamp, T. & Walters, L. (eds) *Contemporary Issues in Bioethics*, 2nd edn. Belmont: Wadsworth.

Harris, E.E. (1966) Respect for persons. In De George, R.T. (ed.) *Ethics and Society*. London: Macmillan.

O'Connor, M.A. (1987) Health/illness and healing/caring – a feminist perspective. In Orr, J. (ed.) *Women's Health in the Community*. Chichester: J. Wiley & Sons.

Orr, J. (ed.) (1987) *Women's Health in the Community*. Chichester: J. Wiley & Sons.

The President's Commission for the Study of Ethical Problems in Medicine and

Biomedical and Behavioural Research (1982) *Making Health Care Decisions.* Washington, DC: US Government Printing Office.

Seedhouse, D. (1988) *Ethics: the Heart of Health Care.* Chichester: J. Wiley & Sons.

Smith, D. (1975) The statistics of mental illness: what they will not tell us about women and why. In *Women Look at Psychiatry.* Vancouver: Vancouver Press Gang.

Smith, J.E. (1967) Autonomy of ethics. In MacQuarrie, J. (ed.) *A Dictionary of Christian Ethics.* Norwich: Fletcher & Son Ltd.

Tingle, J. & Cribb, A. (eds) (1995) *Nursing Law and Ethics.* Oxford: Blackwell Science, pp. 200, 241–243.

Webb, C. (1987) Defining women and their health: the case of hysterectomy. In Orr, J. (ed.) *Women's Health in the Community.* Chichester: J. Wiley & Sons.

Wieczorek, R.R. & Natopoff, J.N. (1981) *A Conceptual Approach to the Nursing of Children,* Philadelphia: Lippincott.

16

The rights of the nurse

For the most part the emphasis so far has been on the rights of the patient and the duties of the nurse towards the patient. When there has been discussion of the rights and responsibilities of the nurse it has been within the context of interpersonal relationships, nurse–patient or nurse–doctor relationships. In this chapter we shall be concerned chiefly with the rights, and to some extent the duties and responsibilities, of the nurse in a wider context. Two further topics are discussed: namely, the relationship between morality and the law, and the value and limitations of professional codes of ethics. The chapter concludes with some thoughts on ethical decision-making.

In Chapter 6 we saw that there are different types of rights – *option rights* and *welfare rights*. We also saw that rights are not unlimited. Restrictions may be imposed, either because the exercise of one's right to do something might impinge upon another right of someone else, or because one also has a duty to behave in a particular way. A nurse, as a human being, shares with all other human beings certain option rights, and as a citizen of a particular society they share with their fellow citizens certain welfare rights.

Now, given that rights are not unlimited, the question is 'Does being a nurse in itself impose limits on any of a person's rights?' The answer is that to some extent it must do. For one reason, in becoming a nurse, a person accepts certain duties. Everyone has a right to health care, although it is a right that we exercise only when we need to – when we become a 'patient'. Nurses, by virtue of their profession, have a duty to enable a patient to exercise that right. The nurse also has a duty to ensure that no harm befalls the patient. There will almost inevitably be occasions when the nurse's rights as an individual will be limited by these two fundamental duties. There may also be occasions when the nurse, in order to fulfil one or both of these duties, will be justified in exercising a personal right to the full. There may be occasions when in order to fulfil that duty to prevent harm to a patient, nurses would be morally justified in exercising their right to act in accordance with their conscience and not comply with another duty, such as the duty to abide by the contract to their employers. For, as we saw in Chapter 6, one is justified in not acting in accordance with one duty in order to comply with another, higher duty.

APPEALS TO CONSCIENCE

'Childress suggests that an appeal to conscience is based on a desire to preserve one's integrity or wholeness as a person' (Benjamin and Curtis, 1992). In making an appeal to conscience one is claiming that to act in a particular way would be a betrayal of one's personal values and beliefs. How one acquires a particular set of values and beliefs is influenced by several factors, as we have seen in the early chapters. One's concepts of right and wrong will be influenced by one's family, culture and religion and also by personal experience. Beliefs are personal and subjective. Thus in saying 'I cannot do that because it is against my conscience', one is saying 'It is wrong for *me*; *I* would feel ashamed; *I* would not be true to myself'. When nurses refuse to carry out a particular procedure on the grounds that it is against their conscience, they are not saying that no nurse should do it. It should be noted that we are here talking about acts which are contrary to an individual's values and beliefs, and not those which could be argued as being contrary to the ethic of the profession.

Generally, it seems, we accept the idea that people have a right to act in accordance with their personal beliefs and values. Henderson (1969) gives as one of her components of basic nursing care: 'Helping the patient practise his religion or conform to his concept of right and wrong.' Henderson's components of nursing care are derived from what she defines as basic human needs. Thus, if to be able to conform to one's concept of right and wrong is a basic human need, then nurses too share that need. A *need* is something which is *felt* or *experienced*, and as such something over which an individual has little control. You cannot stop yourself feeling a need. This applies equally to physical needs, such as hunger, to emotional needs, such as the need to be loved, and to spiritual needs, such as the need to worship.

If we accept the idea that nursing is about helping people to meet those needs which they would meet for themselves if they had the 'necessary strength, will or knowledge', then we have begun to accept the idea that people have a *right* to have those needs met.

The *Universal Declaration of Human Rights* adopted by the United Nations General Assembly in 1948 proclaims that all people have the right to freedom of thought, conscience and religion and to freedom of opinion and expression. Nurses, no less than any other individuals, possess those rights. Nurses therefore have the right to *appeal to conscience*, to refuse to act in such a way that impinges upon their freedom of belief and expression.

The right to make a conscientious objection is acknowledged by the UKCC Code of Professional Conduct, which states: 'As a registered nurse, midwife or health visitor, you ... must: report to an appropriate person or authority, at the earliest possible time, any conscientious objection which may be relevant to your professional practice' (UKCC, 1992).

Having established the principle, we now consider its application.

CONSCIENTIOUS OBJECTION TO ABORTION

Abortion is one procedure to which many nurses hold a conscientious objection. 'Strong and negative attitudes towards patients having elective terminations of pregnancy were expressed by nurses interviewed in a study of gynaecological nurses' attitudes to and opinions of their work' (Webb, 1985). Kemp (1984) found that nurses' attitudes to abortion were significantly affected by religious belief.

The 1967 Abortion Act does allow nurses to be excused from participation in abortions if they have a conscientious objection, but not in all cases. In Kemp's study, the majority of nurses surveyed did not realize that, in emergency situations, nurses are required by law to participate in abortion procedures; the 'conscience clause' cannot be invoked. Kemp concludes that there is a need for greater coverage of all aspects of abortion in nurse training.

Given that, (1) the law in the United Kingdom allows nurses to invoke the conscience clause in most cases and (2) the Code requires nurses to make known any conscientious objection they hold, the problem would seem easily solved. A nurse having registered his or her objection would clearly not choose to work in a situation where abortions were routinely performed. However, the problem is not that simple. Firstly, abortions are frequently carried out, not in separate units or operating theatres, but on a gynaecological ward which provides care for patients with a range of conditions, or within routine gynaecological operating lists. Are nurses who may have a particular interest in gynaecology but who are opposed to abortion to be prevented from pursuing their interest? Secondly, although trained nurses can choose in which speciality they work, nurse learners cannot.

Nurses working on wards or in theatres where abortions form part of the general workload face a dilemma. If they refuse to participate in abortions they may feel that they are placing an additional workload on their colleagues. Their refusal may also cause administrative difficulties about which they may feel uncomfortable. Nurse learners may feel that in refusing to participate in abortions they will miss out on an important part of training. 'Where nurses are ambivalent about abortion, or where they are definitely opposed to it, I think it is extremely important for them to be strong in saying so, and in defending their own moral convictions' (Kenny, 1984). In matters of conscience, if one is to be true to oneself, then it may mean going against the general tide and accepting the consequences.

On the issue of abortion, nurses do not fall into two clearly defined camps: those who on the one hand are opposed to it on principle, and those on the other hand who have no objection to it. Many nurses would say that abortion is permissible in some circumstances but not others.

For example, Benjamin and Curtis (1992) cite a case in which amniocentesis was to be performed in order to identify the gender of the fetus. The nurse involved had come to believe that abortion was justifiable in cases of a fetus which was extremely likely to be born severely mentally handicapped, although she was in most other circumstances opposed to abortion. In the particular case cited, the parents had asked for amniocentesis in order to determine the gender of the child and had made it clear that they intended to request an abortion if the child was male. The doctor involved in the case was prepared to carry out the abortion. The nurse felt the procedure unjustified because she considered that abortion was not justified on these grounds.

The nurse in this situation considered there was a distinction between aborting a perfectly healthy fetus and aborting an unhealthy one. Morally, she had every right to refuse to participate in the procedure on this occasion even though in the past she had willingly consented to participating in abortions.

THE NURSE AS PATIENT'S ADVOCATE

According to the UKCC (1989):

> *Advocacy is concerned with promoting and safeguarding the well-being and interests of patients and clients. It is not concerned with conflict for its own sake. ... Dictionaries define advocate as 'one who pleads the cause of another' or 'one who recommends or urges something' and this indicates that advocacy is a positive, constructive activity.*

In Chapter 1 I argued that advocacy is increasingly being seen as an essential part of the nurse's role, and that one of the main functions of the nurse as patient's advocate is to ensure that their rights are met. The paramount right of patients is to safe and considerate care. They have the right to expect that whatever is done to or for them will be in their best interests.

Where do nurses stand if they feel that patients are being mistreated? Do nurses have the right to speak out on behalf of patients who perhaps are unable to do so for themselves? These are fundamental questions and ones about which nurses seem very uncertain.

Firstly, though, what do we mean by 'mistreated'? It is obviously a term which can include a range of meanings. It includes the failure on the part of professionals and/or institutions to give adequate care, to allow patients their rights – for example, to informed consent, to refuse treatment and so on; the carrying out of unnecessary treatment; and it also includes physical and mental abuse.

The International Code of Nursing Ethics (1973) states: 'The fundamental responsibility of a nurse is to promote health, prevent illness, restore health and alleviate suffering. ... The nurse takes appropriate action to safeguard the individual when his care is endangered by a co-worker or any other person.'

Nurses then have not merely the *right* but also a *responsibility* to act on behalf of the patient if they feel that he or she is being mistreated. However, as several reports in the press and elsewhere have shown, it is not always easy for nurses to take on the role of patient's advocate (Beardshaw, 1981).

The Report of a Committee of Enquiry investigating allegations concerning the care and treatment of patients at St Augustine's Hospital, Canterbury, in 1976 concluded that a degree of force which exceeded legitimate persuasion had been used to administer electroconvulsive therapy (ECT) to unwilling informal patients on many occasions (Beardshaw, 1981). If nurses believe that any treatment is being incorrectly or unnecessarily carried out, then they have (1) a *right* to refuse to participate and (2) a *duty* to make a complaint.

The refusal to participate can be made on the basis that the patient's rights are being undermined or by making an appeal to conscience. If the nurse has reason for believing that, as the Enquiry cited above found, the treatment is being administered against the patient's wishes and that the patient is being coerced into giving consent, then the nurse has a right to refuse to participate. The question of ECT is a very controversial one; its therapeutic value has been questioned (Fromer, 1981). If the therapy used to change or control behaviour involves the infliction of pain or a loss of dignity, then it is even more questionable.

It would seem, then, that a nurse could, and should be able to, refuse to participate in a form of therapy, such as ECT, on the grounds that it is against their conscience.

The refusal by a nurse to participate in certain procedures in general, or in individual cases, is not the end of the matter. The procedure will still in all probability be carried out. The question then is whether the nurse has a right to take it further. As has already been seen, it can be difficult enough for a nurse to refuse to participate in certain procedures. It can be even more difficult for the nurse to take on the role of patient's advocate. Beardshaw found that nurses working in mental hospitals frequently did not make complaints about ill-treatment of patients for several reasons. The main reasons for remaining silent were fear of victimization, fear of cover-ups, and that complaints would achieve nothing.

If, and there seems little doubt that it is so, nurses have a right, indeed a duty, to speak out on behalf of their patients, then the profession, employers and society as a whole have a duty to allow them freedom to exercise that right. There are formal procedures available to nurses to make complaints, but, as Beardshaw discovered, these can be very formidable. Furthermore, nurses are not always aware of their rights or the avenues available to them. If they do initiate a complaint they may not always follow it through if they meet with difficulties and obstructions. 'Staying the course may call for great reserves of stamina and determination particularly if the issues are multiple' (Thorold, 1981).

Suppose that a nurse has evidence of maltreatment of a patient who is unable to take any action themselves. The nurse's first move would be to make a complaint through the management hierarchy to their employing authority. If they feel that the complaint is not dealt with satisfactorily, that no action is taken or the matter is 'hushed up', what further steps can be taken? There are several other channels open to them. They can raise the matter with their professional association or trade union; they can, in the United Kingdom, report it to the Health Service Commissioner; seek the help of the local Community Health Council; or report it to the UKCC. Unfortunately, in pursuing these avenues the nurse may be made to feel disloyal to colleagues or employer. However, these various bodies exist in order to protect the nurse, the patient or both, and nurses have a right, moral and legal, to avail themselves of them.

Complaints officially lodged in any of the ways mentioned may result in a formal enquiry being set up, either an internal enquiry on the part of the Health Authority or a government enquiry. The findings of such enquiries may or may not be made public. The concern is that if enquiry findings are not publicized then little or no action may result. Furthermore, nurses may fear that if findings are published then their hospital will be brought into disrepute, which would reflect upon their own and their colleagues' professional reputations.

The next question is 'Do nurses have the right to draw public attention to cases of malpractice?'

It is curious, given the value that is supposed to be placed on freedom of speech and freedom of the press in Britain, that so many legal doubts remain about the right of an employee to give information to the press.

(Beardshaw, 1981)

As far as the law stands, at least in the way in which it operates in practice, going to the press is a last resort which should only be undertaken if all other official avenues have been exhausted. The nurse who goes to the press is likely to be sanctioned by the law.[1]

This issue, commonly known as *whistle-blowing*, is extremely complex, and the UKCC Code of Conduct is somewhat ambiguous on the subject. While the Code implies that a nurse might have a duty to make known any injustices in health care – 'shall act, at all times, in such a manner as to: serve the interests of society' – it does seem to leave the onus on the individual practitioner. Whereas Clauses 11, 12 and 13 of the Code require the nurse to 'report to an appropriate person or authority' any matters likely to affect patient safety or standards of practice, they do not specify who such appropriate persons or authorities might be. When the Code does make reference to divulging confidential information 'in the wider public interest' (Clause 10), it is the individual practitioner who has to be able to justify such disclosure.

From a purely moral standpoint one could argue that it is in the public interest that information should be made known. The public have a right to know what is going on. Members of the public have a right to know how safe they will be if they submit themselves to the care of the Health Service. Nurses may therefore find themselves in a position where their moral convictions conflict with their legal rights and duties and also possibly with their professional rights. We shall return to this vexed question of morality versus legality later, but first we consider one further issue.

WITHDRAWAL OF LABOUR

Do nurses have a right to withdraw their labour, and would they ever be justified in going on strike? First, let us consider the question as to whether there is a *right to strike*. If such a right exists, then it is a *welfare* right and not a *natural* or *option* right. That is to say that the right to strike cannot be equated with such rights as those to life or to freedom.

The argument that one has a right to strike can be made on the basis of a fundamental right to justice. The right to justice means that one has a right to fair terms of employment, a right to adequate working conditions and to reasonable reward. If one is denied these rights then one has a right to strike in order to obtain them. As far as nurses and other health workers are concerned, however, other fundamental rights have to be taken into account. The patient, indeed the population as a whole, has a right to health care. Inevitably, if nurses exert a right to strike they will restrict the rights of others to health care. Rights cannot be rights if they are exercised at the price of harm to others.

Any industrial action in the Health Service, be it an all-out strike, a work-to-rule or a refusal to deal with nothing other than 'emergencies', will harm patients. It will mean increased waiting time for treatment, delay in diagnosis and a deterioration in standards of care. Patients will therefore suffer. To strike or take any form of industrial action for the purposes of improving pay is morally unjustifiable. Would it though be justifiable in order to improve health care or to prevent harm to patients?

Some have claimed that nurses would be justified in taking industrial action in order to draw attention to, and, it is hoped, rectify, inadequate health care provision. Utilitarians would argue that to strike in order to achieve the end of improved health care was justified, on the grounds that, while some individuals might suffer, the end aimed for was the greater good for the greater number. The argument against this contention is that, while nurses as a whole have a duty towards the population as a whole, they also have individual duties and responsibilities toward individual patients. The nurse's duty towards the individual patient already under their care supersedes the collective duty of all nurses toward the whole population.

If, on the other hand, nurses were ordered by their employer or the government to act in a way which was clearly harmful to patients, then they could be justified in refusing so to do. 'If, for example, under a Nazi Government a policy decision was taken to perform selective euthanasia on demented elderly patients, one would hope nurses would be prepared to strike rather than implement the policy' (Thompson *et al.*, 1983). In less dramatic situations nurses would have to decide whether patients would suffer more because of poor conditions, lack of manpower or resources, or as a result of industrial action.

Another possible justification for withdrawal of labour might be if nurses were required to work in conditions which were harmful to themselves. If, for example, an NHS Trust failed to provide nursing staff with the correct protective clothing or equipment for caring for patients with a highly contagious disease, would the nurses be justified in refusing to care for those patients? Here the nurses would have to balance the risk to their own health against the risks to the patients. Clearly, the onus is on the Trust, indeed on society as a whole, to provide nurses with safe working conditions and the tools to do the job it requires of them. Society does not have the right to expect that nurses should put their own health or lives at risk in order to fulfil their duty to society. In such a situation the decision has to be one for each individual nurse, and those who refuse to work under such circumstances should not be condemned.

MORALITY VERSUS LEGALITY

'Most stable societies have a long tradition of law and custom that embodies the established moral consensus of that society' (Thompson *et al.*, 1983). Thus in many cases what is right or wrong in law may also be right or wrong morally. However, certain acts may be morally, but not legally, wrong, and vice versa. For example, in the United Kingdom, to take one's own life is not illegal, but many would claim that it is morally wrong. The law does not give a moral sanction to act in a particular way.

Again, one might claim that a law is in itself immoral and that one would therefore be morally justified in breaking that law. Throughout history there have been numerous examples of laws which people have felt morally justified in violating. It is the stuff of which martyrs are made. Even in modern times there have been, and are, many examples. Martin Luther King and his followers felt morally justified in violating the law to protest against the immoral race laws in the United States. Apartheid is considered by many to be morally wrong and therefore, it is claimed, people were morally justified in violating the South African laws of apartheid. The argument of some members of Peace Movements is that possession of nuclear weapons is in itself immoral and that one is justified in protesting against their possession even if doing so means violating the law of the land.

Within the context of health care it is easy to envisage extreme circumstances, such as the example of euthanasia under a Nazi Government referred to earlier, in which nurses and other health professionals would be morally justified in breaking or refusing to obey the law. Generally speaking, nurses do not find themselves faced with such clear cut situations. In Chapter 9 it was suggested that compliance with the order of a court of law to divulge information about a patient was morally justified. One could, on the other hand, argue that a nurse would be morally justified, and in some cases have a moral duty, to disobey the court's order and face the legal consequences. In the case of contractual law, nurses would be morally justified in not fulfilling their duty to their employer in order to comply with the higher duty to care for their patients. Again, the nurse might be found guilty in law and have to face the consequences of such action. Moral rights or obligations might *excuse* one from obeying the law, but they do not *suspend* the law.

'There will always be acts that are morally permissible or obligatory, but not legal, and vice versa' (Benjamin and Curtis, 1992). The reasons are basically two-fold; firstly, because the nature of ethical enquiry is such that changing circumstances are constantly causing people to re-evaluate and re-interpret moral values, and secondly because it is impossible to legislate to cover every conceivable situation without imposing unacceptable limitation on personal freedom and privacy. Therefore, while one can argue a strong case that in a reasonably just society one has a prima facie obligation to obey the law, that obligation can be overridden in order to comply with a higher, more stringent moral obligation.

PROFESSIONAL CODES

In essence, there are two types of professional codes. There are *codes of ethics* and *codes of conduct*, and it is important to differentiate between the two. 'A code of ethics is a statement of belief. It is a statement about what the profession believes itself and its purpose to be, and, therefore, embodies a statement of belief about human nature' (Rumbold, 1991). Benjamin and Curtis (1992) contend that codes of professional ethics contain two categories of statement: *statements of creed* and *commandments*. Statements of creed or belief 'affirm professional regard for high ideals of conduct and personally commit members of the profession to honour them, thus constituting a sort of oath of professional conduct' (Benjamin and Curtis, 1992). Thus, in the preamble to the American Nurses' Association (1976) *Code for Nurses* we read: 'The Code for nurses is based on belief about the nature of individuals, nursing, health and society.'

So what, then, is a code of conduct? 'A code of conduct is a framework for behaviour. It is a statement about how the profession considers its members should behave toward clients, society as a whole and each other' (Rumbold, 1991). To make it more explicit: 'A code of conduct is what is says it is – a code of guidance regarding appropriate conduct for a specific group of people carrying out specific actions' (Burnard and Chapman, 1988).

A code of ethics, then, might provide a member of a profession with statements of belief which the profession holds and to which the member is expected to adhere. For codes of ethics to be of any real help to practitioners they have to go one step further, as

Benjamin and Curtis (1992) suggest. They need to include some statements about conduct (or to use Benjamin and Curtis's terminology – *commandments*).

Codes of conduct, on the other hand, are more concerned with how members of a profession should behave. Inevitably, however, codes of conduct tend to be based on ethical principles and contain within them statements of an ethical nature. For example, 'Statements about confidentiality are based on the belief that individuals have a right to privacy. Whereas statements about not bringing the profession into disrepute, although alluding to immoral behaviour, are maintaining the self-interest of the profession in its status' (Rumbold, 1991).

Professional codes serve three main functions. They serve to reassure the public, they provide guidelines for the profession to discipline and regulate its members, and they provide a framework on which individual members can formulate their decisions.

Codes of conduct and/or ethics are usually more to do with *responsibilities* than with *rights* or *duties*. Many codes of nursing begin with a statement about general responsibilities. 'The fundamental responsibility of the nurse is four fold: to promote health, to prevent illness, to restore health and to alleviate suffering' (ICN, 1973). 'The statements of the *Code* and their interpretation provide guidance for conduct and relationships in carrying out nursing responsibilities consistent with the ethical obligations of the profession and quality of nursing care' (ANA, 1976). Exercising responsibility is quite different from acting in accordance with duty. 'The concept is wider than duty which is generally linked to something prescribed, part of a contract. Responsibility is linked to freedom, to goodness and to rightness' (Tschudin, 1986). Thus, exercising professional responsibility means making decisions about what is the right or wrong course of action based upon a calculated outcome. In exercising responsibility the nurse needs in any situation to judge which of alternative actions will most benefit the patient.

Professional codes cannot and do not provide answers to every situation. Clearly, if the intention is that all nurses should read them, then codes of ethics and/or conduct have to be brief and comprehensible. They also have to be *acceptable* to all nurses.

There is then a danger that they will become vague, abstract and so general that they cannot, without significant interpretation, be applied to many specific situations.

On the other hand, if they attempt to be very specific and comprehensive they are likely to not be acceptable to all and will become extremely lengthy and unlikely as a consequence to be read fully by many nurses. It is in any case impossible to write a code which will provide precise answers for any and every situation. However detailed the code, there comes a point when individuals have to make a decision for themselves.

The purpose of professional codes is to enable members of the profession to exercise accountability and responsibility, and not to dictate actions. 'Even the UKCC Code of Professional Conduct which, more than many others, appears in its use of language to be prescriptive ..., allows for considerable freedom in decision-making' (Rumbold, 1991). It does not, for example, take more than a fairly cursory glance at the Code of Conduct to see that in certain situations there might be conflict between two or more of the statements contained within it. One cannot stick rigidly to the letter of the law, as it were, for to do so would leave one in a position of being up an ethical gum tree.

If the opening statements, together with Clause 1 are taken as being overriding, then is it possible to always comply rigidly with Clauses 5 and 6? Clause 10 might also, in some circumstances, pose the individual practitioner with a moral dilemma.

(Rumbold, 1991)

CONCLUSION – MAKING ETHICAL DECISIONS

Ethical decisions, like other professional decisions, should be informed. Many of the ethical issues in nursing and health care are emotive. Most of us approach such issues as abortion, euthanasia and apportioning health funds with strongly felt emotions. The first step in ethical decision-making is to avoid making a purely emotional response.

How, then, should one approach ethical decisions? Firstly, one needs a framework to guide one's thinking. Professional codes of ethics are one aid. A knowledge and understanding of ethical theories are also necessary, not only to provide one with a framework on which to work but also to give one an understanding of how others might approach the subject. The purpose of books such as this one is to enhance knowledge and understanding of ethical theories. Secondly, it is important to be able to argue from a sound knowledge base. This means having a grounding in such areas as the biological and social sciences, the nature and treatment of diseases, and keeping abreast of developments in nursing and nursing research. It also means gathering all the relevant facts pertaining to the specific situation. Thirdly, one needs to be able to argue one's case clearly and logically and avoid leaping to conclusions on the basis of too little or inaccurate information.

No one can withdraw from moral decision-making, and nurses along with members of other professions, because of the nature of their work are faced with making decisions of a moral or ethical nature more frequently than other members of society. The importance for nurses of examining their own beliefs and values and of understanding how they arrived at them cannot be overemphasized. Nor can it be overemphasized that nurses should not seek to impose their own values on either their colleagues or patients. By the same token, no one should allow themselves to be easily swayed by emotive arguments. Perhaps the overriding principle in moral decision-making is *honesty* – honesty towards others but more importantly honesty with and to oneself. 'To thine own self be true' (*Hamlet*).

NOTE

1. For further discussion of this issue, see Thorold, O. (1981) Nurse whistleblowers and the law. In Beardshaw, V. (1981) *Conscientious Objectors at Work*. London: Social Audit.

REFERENCES

American Nursing Association (1976) *Code for Nurses with Interpretative Statements*, ANA.

Bandman, E.L. & Bandman, B. (1990) *Nursing Ethics through the Life Span*. Englewood Cliffs: NJ: Prentice-Hall.

Beardshaw, V. (1981) *Conscientious Objectors at Work*. London: Social Audit.

Benjamin, M. & Curtis, J. (1992) *Ethics in Nursing*, 3rd edn. New York: Oxford University Press.

Burnard, P. & Chapman, C. (1988) *Professional and Ethical Issues in Nursing*. Chichester: J. Wiley & Sons.

Fromer, M.J. (1981) *Ethical Issues in Health Care*. St Louis: C.V. Mosby.

Henderson, V. (1969) *Basic Principles of Nursing Care*. Geneva: ICN.

International Council of Nurses (1973) *Code for Nurses*. Geneva: ICN.

Kemp, J. (1984) Attitudes to abortion. *Nursing Mirror*, 25 April, 158(17), 34–35.

Kenny, M. (1984) All in the Line of Duty? *Nursing Mirror*, 16 May, 158(20), 22–23.

Rumbold, G. (1991) *Ethics in Nursing and Midwifery Practice*. London: Distance Learning Centre, South Bank Polytechnic.

Thompson, I.E., Melia, K.M. & Boyd, K.M. (1983) *Nursing Ethics*. Edinburgh: Churchill Livingstone.

Thorold, O. (1981) Nurse whistleblowers and the law. In Beardshaw, V. (1981) *Conscientious Objectors at Work*. London: Social Audit.

Tschudin, V. (1986) *Ethics in Nursing – the Caring Relationship*. London: Heinemann.

UKCC (United Kingdom Central Council for Nursing, Midwifery and Health Visiting) (1989) *Exercising Accountability*. London: UKCC

UKCC (1992) *Code of Professional Conduct for the Nurse, Midwife and Health Visitor*, 3rd edn. London: UKCC.

Webb, C. (1985) Nurses' attitudes to therapeutic abortion. *Nursing Times*, 2 January, 81(1), 44–47.

FURTHER READING

On appeals to conscience

Benjamin, M. & Curtis, J. (1992) *Ethics in Nursing*, 3rd edn. New York: Oxford University Press.

See references to 'Conscience' and 'Conscientious Refusal'.

Thompson, I.E., Melia, K.M. & Boyd, K.M. (1983) *Nursing Ethics*, Edinburgh: Churchill Livingstone.

See Chapter 3, 'Responsibility and Accountability in Nursing'.

On withdrawal of labour

Benjamin, M. & Curtis, J. (1992) *Ethics in Nursing,* 3rd edn. New York: Oxford University Press.

See references to 'Strikes'.

Thompson, I.E., Melia, K.M. & Boyd, K.M. (1983) *Nursing Ethics.* Edinburgh: Churchill Livingstone.

See Chapter 6, 'Nurses and Society', for a full discussion of this topic.

On morality versus legality

Edwards, P. (ed.) (1967) *Encyclopedia of Philosophy.* New York: Macmillan and Free Press.

See 'Responsibility, Moral and Legal', Kaufman, Arnold S.

Reich, W.J. (1978) *The Encyclopedia of Bioethics.* New York: Macmillan and Free Press.

See 'Law and Morality', Brody, B.A.

Smith, J.P. (1983) The relationship between rights and responsibilities in health care: a dilemma for nurses. *Journal of Advanced Nursing,* 8, 437–440.

Tingle, J. & Cribb, A. (eds) (1995) *Nursing Law and Ethics.* Oxford: Blackwell Science

See: Preface; Chapter 1 'The Legal Dimension', Ann Young; Chapter 2 'The Ethical Dimension', Alan Cribb; and Chapter 5B 'An Ethical Perspective – Negligence and Moral Obligations', Graham C. Rumbold & Harry Lesser.

Thompson, I.E., Melia, K.M. & Boyd, K.M. (1983) *Nursing Ethics.* Edinburgh: Churchill Livingstone.

See Chapter 2, Section 4, on 'Ethics, Law and Religion'.

On codes of ethics

Benjamin, M. & Curtis, J. (1992) *Ethics in Nursing,* 3rd edn. New York: Oxford University Press.

See references to 'Codes'.

Veatch, R.M. (1981) *A Theory of Medical Ethics.* New York: Basic Books.

See Chapter 4. 'The Problems with Professional Physician Ethics'.

For discussion on the UKCC Code of Professional Conduct

Burnard, P. & Chapman, C. (1988) *Professional and Ethical Issues in Nursing.* Chichester: J. Wiley & Sons.

Jones, I.H. (1990) *The Nurse's Code.* Basingstoke: Macmillan.

Tingle, J. & Cribb, A. (eds) (1995) *Nursing Law and Ethics.* Oxford: Blackwell Science

See Chapter 3 'The Professional Dimension', Reg Pyne.

Index